CURT RICHTER

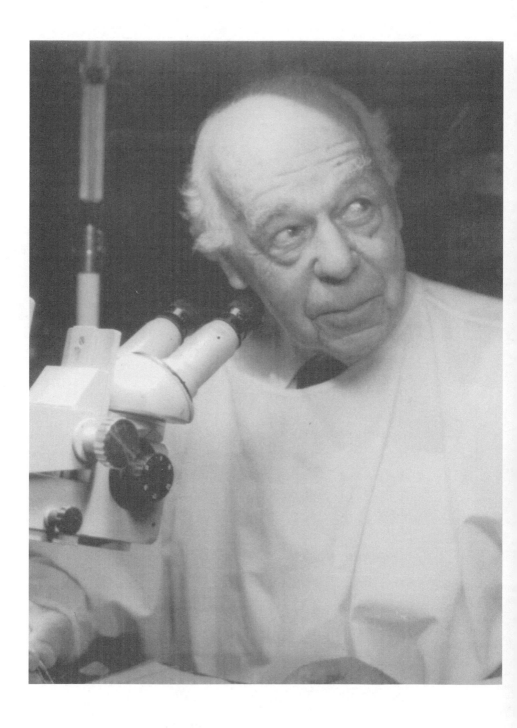

CURT RICHTER

A Life in the Laboratory

JAY SCHULKIN

THE JOHNS HOPKINS UNIVERSITY PRESS

BALTIMORE AND LONDON

© 2005 The Johns Hopkins University Press
All rights reserved. Published 2005
Printed in the United States of America on acid-free paper

2 4 6 8 9 7 5 3 1

The Johns Hopkins University Press
2715 North Charles Street
Baltimore, Maryland 21218-4363
www.press.jhu.edu

Library of Congress Cataloging-in-Publication Data
Schulkin, Jay.
Curt Richter : a life in the laboratory / Jay Schulkin.
p.   ; cm.
Includes bibliographical references and index.
ISBN 0-8018-8073-4 (hardcover : alk. paper)
1. Richter, Curt Paul, 1894–1988. 2. Psychobiology, Experimental—Maryland—Biography.
[DNLM: 1. Richter, Curt Paul, 1894–1988. 2. Behavior—physiology—Biography. 3. Biological
Clocks—Biography. 4. Psychology—Biography. WZ 100 R5356 2005] I. Title
QP360.S366 2005
152'.092—dc22   2004017268

A catalog record for this book is available from the British Library.

Frontispiece: Curt Richter at his microscope (1976). *Source:* Alan Mason Chesney
Medical Archives, Johns Hopkins Medical Institutions

For Alan Rosenwasser, Jon Schull, and Betsy Wood

CONTENTS

FOREWORD

The pictures of my two mentors hang in my office. One is Jean Mayer, my thesis sponsor. The other is Curt Richter, whom I did not meet until after my thesis was complete. But more and more, as the years pass, I realize that Curt Richter has been my model for how to do science, how to be an inquirer. I consider Curt Richter to have been the greatest psychobiologist of the twentieth century. He epitomized the approach of finding "big phenomena" (as my colleague, Philip Teitelbaum, describes them), that is, large, striking effects, which he then explored. Over and over again, he discovered something really important, brought it into the laboratory, tamed it with his ingenuity, amazing engineering ability, and great hands, and shed light on something interesting to us all. Richter's nose for phenomena was his greatest asset. His style was to open scientists' eyes to something we had not appreciated and give us some ideas about how to investigate it. Then, in most cases, he was on to something else. This breadth is apparent from the very beginning of his career. "His first seven papers (1921–25) deal with determinants of spontaneous activity, biological clocks, endocrine control of behavior, the origin of the electrical resistance of the skin, brain control of the motor system, and a device to aid in the measurement of salivation. All these beginnings developed into lifelong interests. . . . The breadth of this total entry into the scientific literature is so great, that none of his first seven papers refer to any of the others!" (Rozin 1976a).

Richter is the quintessential example of what Jay Schulkin calls "a laboratory state of mind." As Eliot Stellar described Richter, "It is hard to imagine the joy of scientific investigation unless you've witnessed it directly. To see curiosity and humbleness go hand in hand, to see unabashed enthusiasm for new ideas, to see excitement over little achievements that inevitably add up to a big picture, to see that weather-eye out for the new shape of understanding, all this is to see Curt Richter" (Stellar 1976, p. xi).

There is very little big theory in the Curt Richter corpus, and not much fancy equipment. His striking effects did not require, and usually did not receive, summary statistics, let alone inferential statistics. He just came up with one winner after another. He understood how to use natural pathologies, reproduced in the laboratory, to illuminate the normal state of affairs. He worked seamlessly across physiological and behavioral analyses, always with an idea of how what he studied was adaptive in an evolutionary sense.

And he worked steadily, and really hard. His career was uninterrupted by moves of his lab from one place to another. Richter did his thesis under John Watson at Johns Hopkins University and stayed there for his whole life. It is hard to imagine anyone more associated with Johns Hopkins.

Richter's major theoretical contribution was the idea of behavioral homeostasis, and he provided a massive amount of evidence for it. He brought ideas about constancy of the internal environment (Claude Bernard) and homeostasis (Walter Cannon) into the realm of behavior and psychology.

Richter is like the proverbial elephant explored by small creatures standing on its surface. Few, other than Jay Schulkin, have the full picture. Is it the *same* Richter who invented the activity wheel, pioneered the studies of food self-selection and biological clocks, and studied inhibitory reflexes, taste, domestication, and sudden death? Yes, it is.

Richter is vastly underappreciated for several reasons, not least because he worked on such a broad set of problems. Individuals usually become famous because a lifetime of excellent work connects their name to some major advance, but Curt worked on too many things to make enough of a mark in any one, with the exception of behavioral homeostasis. His genius was spread across three disciplines: physiology, animal behavior/evolutionary biology, and psychology, and this created another intellectual dilution effect. Also, his focus was almost entirely on collecting data and reporting it; he wrote relatively few reviews and made almost no attempts to reach a broad psychology and biology audience. He had very few students because he was a professor in a medical school as opposed to a Ph.D.-granting department, and this in the days before postdoctoral fellowships were common. His influence was through the colleagues he inspired, including Eliot Stellar, Philip Teitelbaum, Alan Epstein, Jay Schulkin, and me.

I have tried, in my modest way, to find big phenomena and to open up new views and opportunities for our enterprise. I am in Richter's shadow, but I am glad to be there and to have been inspired by him.

Richter is a great and unique inquirer. And this book about him is written by another very special inquirer. Jay Schulkin's natural link to Richter is their common interest in mineral appetites, particularly sodium and calcium. Richter was the pioneer in this area, and Schulkin is an eminent student of these phenomena today. Indeed, he has written two books on the subject.

But there are other parallels between these two scientists. Richter was a poor student as an undergraduate at Harvard, someone who did not thrive in the lecture-exam framework, who went at his own pace, and who took off when he had a lab to work with under John Watson. (According to Richter, Watson left him alone and told him to go into the lab and find something interesting. Richter did, producing in 1921 a classic thesis on activity rhythms in rats.) Jay Schulkin was also a nontraditional student. He left high school before graduating and studied with George Wolf at SUNY Purchase College, performing some promising research. I first met him when he came to the University of Pennsylvania to see about graduate work there. He wasn't just a student in the narrow sense of the word but quintessentially a student, an inquirer in the broader sense. Watson let Curt Richter fly, and it was Eliot Stellar who let Jay fly in the anatomy department at Penn. Eliot tailor-made the curriculum for Jay, so he could go through without taking all the academic steps that are usually requisite. And Eliot was rewarded with some first-rate research and colleagueship.

Jay collaborated with more colleagues at Penn than anyone I can remember. He coauthored papers with Eliot Stellar, Alan Epstein, Harvey Grill, John Sabini, Jon Baron, and me. Here he departs from Richter. But both were turned off by the classroom and turned on by the lab (Richter) or the world of ideas (Schulkin). Richter continued on as a magnificent loner, with few collaborators at his academic level. Jay is most at home playing with ideas with his colleagues. His empirical work is mostly with collaborators, but his remarkable philosophical ventures and syntheses of literatures are done on his own. Neither had many students. Curt Richter's reprint folder in my file cabinets is one of my thickest. Jay Schulkin occupies a linear space on my bookshelves that few others can equal. I look up right now and see eight books, from an edited volume in 1989 to a book called *Rethinking Homeostasis* (what could be more about Richter!) in 2003. And now the present book, on Richter himself. Five of the Schulkin books on my shelf are inspired by Curt Richter.

What a natural combination this book is. What a treat for us all, as one delightful oddball tells us about the biggest and best of the twentieth century's oddballs in psychology. The book is the definitive analysis of the contribution and the man, a true labor of love. The great scope of Richter's contribution is available in only two places: the book edited by Eliot Blass, *The Psychobiology of Curt Richter* (1976), and this more thorough, personal, and biographical account. They don't make them like Curt Richter any more. They never did.

Paul Rozin
Edmund J. and Louise W. Kahn Professor of Psychology
University of Pennsylvania

PREFACE

Curt Richter has been a presence in my life for thirty years. As an undergraduate in the early 1970s, I studied with George Wolf, who introduced me to Richter and his work. Wolf's appreciation for Richter led to my first project in science: a study of mineralocorticoid-induced sodium appetite. As I was about to embark on graduate school, I wrote to Richter about my research, informed him that I would be attending a conference in the Baltimore area, and asked him if I could visit with him. He wrote back and invited me to his laboratory for a visit.

When I moved to Penn as a graduate student, the combined presence of Alan Epstein, Paul Rozin, and Eliot Stellar only heightened my appreciation for Richter. They truly admired the man. Each had worked on the biological basis of specific hungers and had had much contact with Richter. During this period, I made several visits to Richter's laboratory. He was always gracious and would say, slightly seductively, "I want you to talk slowly so I can understand everything you are saying." He wanted you to know he was paying attention.

After Richter died, in 1988, I began to write about him. I wrote two pieces immediately after his death, one for the journal *Psychobiology* (Schulkin 1989) and the other, with my senior colleagues Paul Rozin and Eliot Stellar, for the National Academy of Sciences (Schulkin, Rozin, and Stellar 1994). Then came a piece on Richter with my colleague Timothy Moran for the *American Journal of Physiology* (Moran and Schulkin 2000).

A one-day conference held at Johns Hopkins in 1996 put me in touch with others who were interested in Richter's work. It was attended by Daniel Todes and F. L. Holmes (both historians of science), Paul McHugh (Richter's last chairman), and other individuals interested in Richter or his laboratory material. Many of us gave small presentations. My talk placed Richter in the context of Benjamin Franklin, the American pragmatists, and the culture of invention and open-ended inquiry. Richter (1953f) pursued open-ended inquiry that was knotted to invention and experimentation and revealed diverse forms of self-regulatory behaviors that aided successful behavioral adaptation. Richter was an exemplar of a *laboratory state of mind.*

When Richter died, Paul McHugh and Eliot Stellar (see Stellar files, University of Pennsylvania Archives) ensured that the Richter material (e.g., charts, data, personal papers) would be preserved. It was decided that Hopkins would house the Richter archives.

Elliott Blass edited a volume of Richter's work that appeared in 1976. This is a very important book for anyone interested in Richter's work, and the only one in which many of Richter's papers are collected. The introductory essays by Derek Denton, Paul Rozin, and Eliot Stellar in that volume provide an orientation to Richter's scientific work and to Richter the scientist.

The resources used in the preparation of this book included collections of unpublished writings from scholarly archives, references to which appear throughout the text. These include the Alan Mason Chesney Medical Archives at the Johns Hopkins University School of Medicine (www.medicalarchives .jhmi.edu). The archives' holdings include a variety of material from Richter. Throughout I have referenced these materials with the notation "Chesney Archives." Medical archivists Nancy McCall and Marjorie Kehoe and their colleagues have played a vital role in preserving and cultivating the use of Richter's papers and research data and have been very helpful to me.

Other archival sources include interviews conducted by Anne Roe, who collected data on sixty-four scientists for her book *The Making of a Scientist* (Roe 1953). Roe collected transcripts of interviews, personal data, and letters from these scientists, including Richter. These materials, now included in the archives of the American Philosophical Society, are cited with the notation "Roe interviews, American Philosophical Society Archives." Finally, archives of the University of Pennsylvania also contain information pertaining to Richter. I refer to these papers with the notation "University of Pennsylvania Archives."

This book is intended to renew discussion of Richter's work and his orientation to research. Curt Richter is not well known. Why? He had no students. He was not in a psychology department; he was sequestered in a clinic in a medical school. He avoided committees. And he was mainly someone who demonstrated phenomena and did little grand theorizing.

THE STRUCTURE OF THE BOOK

This book examines Richter's personal experience, his orientation to psychobiological research, the intellectual and personal influences in his life, his varied research topics (which form the bulk of the book), and his laboratory and methodological contributions to science. Chapter 1 provides a background account of Richter's personal history, his intellectual trajectory, and some primary influences on his experimental outlook. Chapter 2 discusses the research orientation that Richter maintained over sixty-some years—I refer to his research on biological clocks, their diverse forms, and their expression in both adaptation and disease. Amid the debates of whether psychology could be a science, Richter demonstrated a science of behavior, beginning with studies on the biological basis of behavioral activity and inactivity. Chapter 3 discusses the range of research findings on the role of behavior and physiology in serving the body's nutritional requirements. No concept was more important for Richter than that of homeostasis, or "the wisdom of the body" (Starling 1923; Cannon 1932/1966), in relation to the many systems he explored that help maintain nutritional balance. But behavioral regulation of the internal milieu is understood in relation to the concept of instinct, which played a vital role in organizing Richter's orientation to psychobiological adaptation.

Chapter 4 discusses a concern of primary interest since Darwin, the effect of domestication on end-organ systems. This was an important research theme for Richter. Equally important was his intriguing research on wild rats' bait shyness, poisoning, taste avoidance, and sudden death. Chapter 5 describes a trip Richter made to Panama that resulted in a set of long-term neurological investigations that had clinical implications. The study centered on the neurological control of motor reflexes, and the clinical tools that emerged would be used to discern neurological damage in humans.

Chapter 6 describes the social milieu in which Richter ran his laboratory and the loyalty of a number of people that worked for or with him over a long period. Richter prided himself on the creation of his laboratory culture, his scientific esthetic, and his surgical innovations. Science cannot exist separately from the individuals who participate in the production of knowledge, Richter included.

The conclusion focuses on the man, what he found, his style of research, and his standing in and contributions to the field of psychobiology. At an international conference on the concept of instinct, Richter presented many of his fundamental contributions. But in an intellectual milieu that was highly charged over the concept of instinct, Richter would remain, as he always seemed, close to the findings that emanated from his laboratory, not the intellectual issues that presupposed his framework.

The epilogue discusses Richter's uniqueness in American psychobiology. His personal legacy is linked to his laboratory sensibility, the richness of his experiments, and his admirable sense of exploration.

≡ ≡ ≡ ≡ ≡

Many individuals across diverse fields have been influenced, directly or indirectly, by Richter's work. The citations in this book to many investigators who have been affected by Richter are limited. I apologize to any who feel left out.

Many of Richter's friends, acquaintances, family members (including two of his children), and colleagues have conversed with me about him and about the fields in which Richter participated. So much in scholarship and experiment rests on mutual support among colleagues. Thank you. I also wish to express appreciation to James Wirth, for his telephone companionship throughout the duration of this project, and to Wendy Harris, of the Johns Hopkins University Press, for her encouragement, support, and suggestions.

CURT RICHTER

Introduction

Curt Richter's is not a household name. He is little known to the general public and, though a psychologist, is probably not known to most psychologists. He was an investigator of behavior and physiology who made profound contributions to our understanding of the behavioral and physiological systems that serve adaptation and long-term viability. Curt Richter was the paradigm of the psychobiological investigator.

In the late 1990s, I spent some time with Timothy Moran at the Alan Mason Chesney Medical Archives at Johns Hopkins poring over some of Richter's laboratory books. We had to wear lead-protective suits that covered us from head to toe to keep us safe from the lead-infested notebooks. Richter's laboratory dated back more than sixty years and lead paint had peeled off the walls and fallen onto his charts. As we looked through the laboratory books, we found nothing that we thought he had not already published (log books on sodium, calcium, and metabolic ingestion), but we were both struck by the beauty of his books—the annotations in the margins, the precision and artistry of his notes. We focused on the nutritional experiments. Notes and drawings, amid carefully collected data, were integral parts of these laboratory artifacts. Despite the age of the books and charts, the care Richter took and the clarity of the records were obvious. Moran and I were filled with awe and appreciation. We were also struck by the economy of his style—he wasted very little.

Just who was Curt Richter? What was the context for his approach to research? He was biological in his understanding of behavior. He was fearless as a scientist-adventurer, and in expression he was always close to an engineer, replete with artisan's sensibilities.

In gaining a sense of Richter, two factors are important: (1) The medical school at Johns Hopkins was an ideal place for him. (2) He was a paradigmatic laboratory researcher.

A CULTURE DEVOTED TO RESEARCH, MEDICAL TREATMENT, AND TEACHING: THE JOHNS HOPKINS UNIVERSITY

After receiving his bachelor's degree from Harvard, Richter pursued a graduate degree in psychology at Johns Hopkins. There he entered a cultural atmosphere devoted to research and intellectual freedom (Gilman 1906), two themes on which Hopkins and its trustees prided themselves (Hawkins 1960).

In the 1870s, Hopkins attracted some of the best minds to Baltimore, including C. S. Peirce, founder and developer of American pragmatism, who was a logician and the son of Benjamin Peirce, the great Harvard mathematician and one of the founders of the National Academy of Sciences (Brendt 1993). "Freedom of research" was a much-used dictum by Daniel Coit Gilman (1906), the first president of Hopkins, and also by Richter (1953f).

Reflecting on his experience at Hopkins, founded in 1878, Richter recalled that Gilman "had inspired many very capable young men to join the academic and medical part of the university, and has inspired those men with high ideas of research and particularly of the freedom of research" (Richter 1985, p. 370). Freedom of inquiry was the cornerstone of Richter's own scientific sensibility (Richter 1953f).

Richter lived his intellectual life in the culture of a hospital, a medical world; it was also a culture of research and teaching. The university and hospital were fresh with youth and full of promise. Outstanding figures such as William Halsted, William Osler, and, later, Harvey Cushing were part of the intellectual medical ambiance (Crowe 1957; Harvey et al. 1989). Hopkins was a relatively new institution; the university had been established less than fifty years before Richter arrived. The Phipps Clinic, the new psychiatric unit at Hopkins, was half a decade old (Harvey et al. 1989).

The philosophy at the medical school was expressed by Claude Bernard, the great French experimental physiologist: "Our single aim is and has always been to help make the well-known principles of the experimental method pervade medical science" (Bernard 1865/1957, p. 3). Bernard, along with Walter Cannon, who was well known for his work on homeostatic regulation and physiological adaptation, had a profound influence on Richter, who would extend their ideas by demonstrating the role of behavior in the regulation of the internal milieu.

Bernard expressed a philosophy of experimental medicine, and the experiment as it relates to theory would figure importantly in Richter's work (see introduction by Henderson in Bernard 1865/1957; Holmes 1974). Richter's two main influences, Bernard and Cannon, elegantly demonstrated the physiological analysis of basic regulatory events. One key issue for Bernard and, later, for Cannon (and certainly, as we will see, for Richter) was keeping the internal milieu stable and functioning (Wolfe, Barger, and Benison 2000).

A concept of the organism as adapting and coping with its environment, formulated by diverse thinkers and culminating in Darwin's great works, was part of the experimental framework of the laboratory cultures that were emerging. But while Bernard was arguing for the fixed nature of biological expression and his science was rooted in methodological considerations, others were trying to conceptualize a more broadly organismic sensibility in which to understand the role of physiological adaptation (e.g., Cannon 1932/1966; Cross and Albury 1987) and, eventually, behavioral adaptation (Richter 1943) in the regulation of the internal milieu.

This experimental ambiance contributed to and helped set the stage for a report by Abraham Flexner (1910/1978), now commonly referred to as the Flexner Report, which was commissioned by the Carnegie Foundation. Flexner asserted that "if, then, a laboratory is a place constructed for the express purpose of facilitating the collection of data bearing on definite problems and the initiation of practical measures looking to their solution, the hospital and the dispensary are laboratories in the strictest sense of the term" (Flexner 1910/1978, p. 92).

The Flexner Report examined the state of medical education at the time and made recommendations for the teaching of laboratory skills and other skills essential for physicians. Physicians needed to be familiar with the workings of the laboratory and exposed to the methods of the biological sciences. But Flexner also noted that the "laboratory method in medicine is considerably less than 100 years old" (Flexner 1910/1978, p. 62). The stated goal of the report was to enhance medical education and the training of physicians by linking the practice of research to medical training; physicians would be under the rubric of science, self-corrective inquiry, scholarly endeavors, and so on (Hudson 1972).[1] Hopkins provided an example of the research-oriented hospital for the rest of the country, showing how a university and teaching hospital were to instruct physicians while caring for patients (Chesney 1943, 1963).[2]

The great bulk of individuals working in Richter's laboratories were medical students (see chapter 6). There they were exposed to the workings of science, and although many of them would not have a career in it, science—the testing of hypotheses, the self-corrective method, the actual doing of experiments—would be part of their sense of who they were. The laboratory sense of science was not foreign to them.

The United States was emerging as an important part of the culture of science; science was to be promoted (Numbers and Rosenberg 1996). There was an abiding faith in science and in scientific education in the United States (Rosenberg 1976/1997), and nowhere was this better represented than at the Johns Hopkins University. The hospital was to be a culture in which research would inform medical decision making. Of course, the experimental physiologists (e.g., Bernard) understood that the end point of their research was to better the human condition by applying what they learned to the practical affairs of human health and well-being.

Richter was fortunate to have fallen in with Adolf Meyer, who was to play a fundamental role in his career. Meyer's name appears often in this book. He was the chair of psychiatry at Hopkins for more than thirty years (until 1941); he embraced American pragmatism and wrote extensively about it, wrote some of the first works on psychobiology, and was erudite in and understood a vast array of sciences. He was also a physician who was devoted to patients and their well-being.

A LABORATORY STATE OF MIND

Richter was glued to his laboratory, and that relationship was a work of beauty—fearless, experimental beauty. He was methodologically driven and held a few core ideas, some of which, including total self-regulation of the internal milieu, he inherited from Darwin, Bernard, Charles Sherrington, Cannon, and Meyer.

His science should be understood against the background of the social environment in which he lived, the scientific paradigms he understood and participated in and expanded upon, and his experimental inventiveness. Science is known in part by the hypotheses it generates (Peirce 1898/1992; Hanson 1971), the paradigms and research orientations in which scientists labor (Kuhn 1962), the methodological innovations that support the everyday practice of science, and the experiments, of course (Galison 1987). Science is a social process; scientists work within frameworks that guide their research, in schools of thought that underlie what they look for and see. Richter was no different from other scientists in this regard.

Richter is best known for his methodological innovations in the laboratory, the way he extended core ideas (e.g., the role of biological clocks in the organization of behavior, the role of behavior in the regulation of the internal milieu), his fearless sense of inquiry, his tenacity in staying with core issues over a lifetime, and his laboratory artistry. He presupposed, like all thinkers, ideas or working hypotheses that guided his investigations. He spent most of his life demonstrating phenomena rather than in the engagement of ideas.

The laboratory culture in which Richter operated assumed a set of psychobiological concepts that were small in number but rich in scope. The field of psychobiology was relatively new; William James (1887, 1890/1952), following Darwin (1859/1965, 1872/1998), pointed to the role of biology in behavioral adaptation, and Adolf Meyer wrote extensively on psychobiology (Meyer 1915). The relationship between psychology and medicine was already part of the discussion of leading scholars, including Robert Yerkes (1921), who was one of Richter's undergraduate teachers (see chapter 1). The concept of psychobiology would take on diverse meanings (see Dewsbury 1991); Richter would become a major proponent of, and would come to represent, psychobiological research.

Richter's laboratory sensibility was replete with wonder and play, and the longevity of his career (more than sixty years) perhaps was linked to this feature. Playfulness was also behind his sense that what mattered was "free research," research institutions and funding agencies that allowed valued individuals great latitude in what they could do, what they could explore (see Richter 1953f). His mode of research discovery was motivated less by experimental design worked out in advance than by open-ended exploration. Richter, like other successful scientists of his day (and our own), was supported by foundations devoted to advancing research in American universities (Kohler 1991).

Some core themes and influences are evident in Richter's contributions. Behavioral regulation and physiological regulation were core themes for Richter. Although exploratory, Richter's approach to research was systematic, inventive, and innovative, yet it had no statistical design. He was like many other investigators in that regard. Richter's approach to the behavioral sciences was a search for innate organization. And although his work was situated in the laboratory, he identified himself as a zoologist (Roe interviews, American Philosophical Society Archives, 1952), or what I call a laboratory ethologist. What do I mean by that term? During Richter's time, the ethologist emphasized innate structure, while the psychologist tended to emphasize learning. There was little room in Richter's understanding of psychobiological events for theories of learning. Richter thought as an engineer (how do you make something?); as a psychobiologist, he was determining the hardware necessary for adaptation. He never strayed far from this perspective.

CHAPTER 1

Origins and Orientations

EARLY INFLUENCES

Curt Richter's *vita,* as written by him for his dissertation, reads: "Curt P. Richter was born February 20, 1894, in Denver, Colorado. He attended the Public Schools in Denver up to the time of his graduation from High School in 1912. The next three years he spent in Germany, chiefly in Dresden. During the greater part of this time he attended the Dresden Technische Hochschule. In 1915 he returned to America and entered Harvard, where he graduated in 1917. During the last year at Harvard he acted as Student-Assistant in the department of Philosophy and Psychology. The next two years were spent in the Army. In January he entered Johns Hopkins University" (Richter 1921).

Curt Richter's parents were newly arrived from the Saxony region of Germany when Richter was born. His father, an iron manufacturer, died in a hunting accident while Richter was still quite young. Newspaper reports said that he was killed by a friend; the headline in the paper read: "P. Richter, Iron Manufacturer, Suddenly Slain by Discharge of His Companion's Gun" (Chesney Archives).

Curt Richter remained an only child. The letters in his file in the Chesney Medical Archives at Johns Hopkins indicate that he was close to his mother throughout her life. She was a strong woman who ran the iron factory after her husband's death. Richter recalled that he took care of himself early on, spending long periods alone. Years later, an interviewer noted that "he [Richter] says he was very close to his mother" (Roe interviews, American Philosophical Society Archives, 1952).

Richter received support from his mother, who appears to have been helpful during the early period of his career and during his divorce from his first wife, Phyllis Greenacre, who became a noted psychoanalyst. This early period was a trying time for Richter, and he turned to his mother for sympathy and encouragement. In the early 1930s, feeling the dual pressures of running a laboratory and going through a divorce, he wrote his mother (in one of many letters to her during this period), "I feel all tired out." Of the divorce and his estranged wife, he told his mother, "I will fight her to the end." In other letters he wrote further about the strain of running his laboratory and staying on top of things in the laboratory. He needed rest. He admitted, in a bout of existential angst, "I don't know what to do" (Chesney Archives, 1930). This correspondence reveals that Richter shared very personal aspects of his life with his mother. He often signed the letters, "with love."

The early experience in his parents' factory never left him. As Richter described in an autobiographical essay, he grew up "learning about tools and machines" during the long hours that he spent in the factory. He described this activity as "play" and himself as fascinated by all kinds of gadgets; he had begun to experiment at a young age (Richter 1985). Moreover, as Richter recalled of his childhood, "I spent a lot of time working on locks and clocks—taking them apart and putting them back together again." Richter called this his "play period," and it was interrupted by the shock of his father's death, resuming only after 1919 (Richter 1985, p. 359).

By all accounts, Richter was gregarious. His high school class portrait depicts him as a participant in many activities. Richter formed a key relationship in high school with the head of his school, Dr. W. Smiley, who had attended Harvard and who took a special interest in Richter. Richter commented: "We formed a close relationship that undoubtedly had much to do with my going to Harvard" (Richter 1985, p. 361). Curt Richter, in need of a father figure, perhaps found one in Dr. Smiley. He would find another some years later at Hopkins.

In Denver, Richter attended public schools and, by his own admission, was never a good student. He excelled in sports, a proficiency that would last a lifetime. Years later, he would be a legendary tennis player at Hopkins, and he was known for his general athletic prowess, including for vaulting over fences when in his seventies (Stellar 1989). Growing up in the West, he worked on farms in the summer and loved hunting. He would later be fearless in the laboratory; for example, he caught wild rats in Baltimore and brought them into the laboratory (see chapter 4).

After graduating from high school, Richter, following what he remembered from childhood to be his father's desire, enrolled at an engineering school in

Germany. He remained at the Technische Hochschule in Dresden for three years, from 1912 to 1915. During this period, Richter had an opportunity to get acquainted with relatives and to spend time with his grandmother in the town from which both of his parents had emigrated. At the engineering school, Richter again excelled in sports. He recalled that "the track season later in the spring and early summer gave me an opportunity to shine as an American" (Richter 1985, p. 363). But war was on the horizon, and the culture shifted. Being an American now rendered Richter vulnerable to abuse in Germany. He described one incident: "Four burly Germans approached me with raised canes and started shouting 'spy'" (Richter 1985, p. 365).

Reflecting later on his experience at the engineering school, Richter said, "Looking back on my work at the Hochschule, I have come to realize how much I learned that has helped me in the running of my Laboratory of Psychobiological Research. Certainly, the experience gained from making the many charts and graphs used in mechanics helped me in many ways in working up results in my biological studies" (Richter 1985, p. 365). On the other hand, he lamented that he was not allowed to do his own experiments at the school, and he still had not taken any courses in biology.

Soon after Richter's return to the United States, he entered Harvard College on the recommendation of his high school mentor, Dr. Smiley, with whom he was still close. At Harvard, by Richter's own admission, he remained a mediocre student. He failed several subjects. His grades were so bad that he was put on probation. Richter said that he excelled in no particular subject until he took a course in genetics, followed by one on the philosophy of nature with E. B. Holt (a student of William James), who throughout his career retained James's sense of psychobiology and his philosophy of nature (see Holt 1931/1976, 1937). Holt came to Richter's defense by writing a letter (dated February 24, 1917) to the assistant dean of Harvard College, Mr. Little, which stated that Richter was "a man of marked ability" and that in Germany Richter had not been exposed to the American method of taking exams, which could account for his poor grades. Holt described Richter as "a very able chap" and expressed an interest in having Richter as his assistant the following year.

Richter (1985) noted that Holt introduced him to Freud's writings; perhaps this included Freud's work on the biological basis of drives. Maybe Richter's career-long interest in the biological embodiment of the concept of drive (McHugh and Slavney 1998) was kindled by this early reading of Freud. Holt was obviously an important person for the young Curt Richter.

Richter noted in the Roe interview that he "got a good grade in a course with Perry"—a student, biographer, and major exponent of the work of William James (Perry 1935)—and that Holt's course "stimulated me to sign up for a short experimental course on insect behavior, given by Professor Robert Yerkes. This course, though short, made me feel that at last I had found something that really interested me. Further, Yerkes thought that I had done quite well and gave me an A in this course, the only A that I ever managed to get during my two years at Harvard, or for that matter, elsewhere" (Richter 1985, p. 369). I could find no correspondence between the two men, and Richter said very little about Yerkes in his autobiographical material, but Yerkes's sense of the importance of the biological basis of behavior (Yerkes 1913) and the study of instinctive behaviors (Yerkes 1930), in addition to the relationship of biology to medicine (Yerkes 1921), no doubt influenced Richter for a lifetime.

Richter described his time in Cambridge as "very interesting but not a happy time"; he was in "mild depression much of the time" (Richter 1985, p. 369). This is not surprising because he often was not doing well in school. Through Holt Richter was introduced to L. J. Henderson (Roe interviews, American Philosophical Society Archives). He had the "good fortune to be invited to have lunch with L. J. Henderson" (Richter 1985, p. 369). He had a great deal of contact with Henderson and said, "Henderson stimulated me more from the physiological side" (Roe interviews, American Philosophical Society Archives). Henderson, a colleague of Walter Cannon's at Harvard and the founder of the Society of Fellows, was very interested in promoting a culture of research within the medical community (Henderson 1935, 1970) and was a basic physiologist with broad interests. An early exponent of the experimental method in physiology and medicine,[1] he wrote an introduction to Claude Bernard's important book on the subject.

Richter noted that his war service was an uneventful tour of duty in the States, highlighted by a visit from Professor Henderson, who "brought me a number of books" (Richter 1985, p. 370). Henderson must have seen the promise in Curt Richter.

J. B. WATSON

On the advice of Yerkes, Richter descended on the city of Baltimore and the Johns Hopkins University. John Watson, the noted behaviorist, had already moved from the Psychology Department at Hopkins to the Phipps Psychiatric

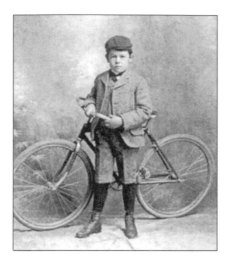

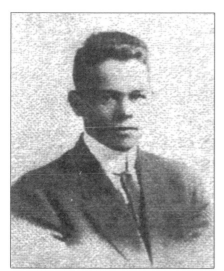 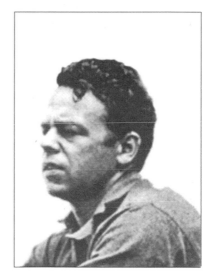

FIG. 1.1. Curt Richter as a young boy (1905), young man (1912), and young scientist (1930). *Source:* Alan Mason Chesney Medical Archives, Johns Hopkins Medical Institutions

Clinic (a part of Hopkins Hospital) when Richter arrived in 1918. Richter knew little about Watson, although he had read Watson's book on animal behavior while still an undergraduate at Harvard (University of Akron Psychology Archives, August 1963). Reflecting on his time as an undergraduate at Harvard, Richter recalled, "Yerkes recommended that I read a book, *Animal*

Behavior, by John B. Watson. After having read only snatches here and there, I became convinced that I should try to work with him. . . . I must point out here that at that time, and for a long time later, I had no idea about what Watson meant by 'behaviorism.' For me 'behaviorism' simply meant 'behavioral'" (Richter 1985, p. 369).

Richter recalled Watson's uttering these words: "I want you to know that I am only interested in getting a good piece of research. You do not have to take any course or attend any lectures. You are strictly on your own" (Richter 1985, p. 371). From that meeting, Richter took away a great feeling of excitement.

Watson, however, had a missionary zeal for behaviorism, the objective measurement of behavior, and, in particular, of reflexive behaviors and conditioning (Boakes 1984; O'Donnell 1985; Benjamin 1988). He believed behaviorism could reform the world, setting psychology straight and firm within "positive knowledge" (positivism). Behaviorism, for Watson, clarified psychologists' thinking. Watson's earlier work was much more rooted in biology than was his later, more well-known material on the study of behavior. His intellectual drive was rigor; his desired goal was scientific respectability. Watson was on an ideological mission to legitimate a science.

Watson had been a graduate student at Chicago,[2] writing a thesis entitled "Animal Education," and he was influenced by J. R. Angell (known for a biological and functionalist perspective) and Henry H. Donaldson (who had been a student at Hopkins) (Watson 1930; Angell et al. 1896; Boakes 1984). In fact, Donaldson wrote an important book that influenced Richter's later research, *The Rat* (Donaldson 1915), which provided normative data on the growth curves of rats and revealed the effects of domestication on end-organ systems (see chapter 4).

While Watson was a student at Chicago, he learned from Donaldson something about what he called "exactness in research" (Watson 1930/1961). And Donaldson influenced some of the work of Richter, namely, his research on the effects of domestication. In an interview, Richter said, "I knew Dr. Henry H. Donaldson quite well. He wrote a well-known book, *The Rat.* . . . Several times a year I met with him" (University of Akron Psychology Archives, 1963). This book was an intellectual point of contact for Richter. Years later, toward the end of Richter's life, he drafted some notes for a paper that he never finished, which was to be a defense of the use of the common rat in animal experimentation.

Watson also provided Richter, in their short time together at Hopkins, with the intellectual freedom that was of the highest value for Richter in that culture of research, with its emphasis on the measurement of behavior. Richter sought in his study of behavior some objective measurement; there was, at the time, no ideology of behavioral analysis remotely close to the Richter concept of research.

Outside of the laboratory, Watson was a legendary party animal both during his time at Hopkins and thereafter (Buckley 1989). Watson would recall being particularly close to both Richter and Karl Lashley (Watson 1930/1961). Richter had a real fondness for Watson personally. He spent time socializing with Watson and visited him in New York for many years after Watson moved there and went into the advertising field. Richter said that Watson and his second wife "entertained almost every single night. I don't see how they took it. No matter how late it was, he stayed up. He was always up on deck the next morning" (University of Akron Psychology Archives, August 1963).

Most importantly, Watson provided Richter the freedom for inquiry that he required and reinforced Richter's enthusiasm for science. Johns Hopkins was now his home.

A CAREER SET IN MOTION

Richter's dissertation, "The Behavior of the Rat: A Study of General and Specific Activities" (Richter 1921), planted the seed for a career in research. It was an attempt to study spontaneous and self-generated behaviors. In contrast with Watson's work, in which behavior was understood as externally caused, Richter's thesis highlighted internally generated behavioral control systems (Rozin 1976a). Richter began with a description of the history of the rat, explained why the rat was a good model for laboratory study, and proceeded to demonstrate how to measure laboratory rat behaviors. He began his dissertation with the bold assertion that "this investigation concerns itself with the general question of finding out how a certain organism, the rat, 'works.'"

His committee included Knight Dunlap, chair of the Department of Psychology, who several years previously had published a book on psychobiology. Dunlap, along with Baldwin, had been instrumental in bringing Watson to Hopkins, and Dunlap took over the position of department chair after Watson's departure to the Department of Psychiatry at the Phipps Clinic (Pauly 1979). Dunlap's book on psychobiology contained virtually nothing on the behavioral component of biological regulation. This would await the work of Richter.

Let us put Richter in perspective: as his career continued at Hopkins, he was a researcher, not a university professor in the current sense. He occasionally taught courses to medical students, usually with someone else. For example, for the Psychobiological Course in 1927, Richter lectured on drive, affect, sleep, and dreams. Adolf Meyer, with whom he was teaching the course, lectured on personality, different views of psychobiology, thinking and memory, sex, and social behavior (Meyer files, Chesney Archives).

In a letter to Meyer dated August 16, 1930, Richter outlined what he called his general topics of investigation. They included skin resistance and psychogalvanic reflex, the pituitary and the third ventricle, spontaneous activity, voluntary and reflex grasping and hanging, anxiety attacks, the experimental production of various emotion states, and depression. Many of these issues would be common avenues of inquiry throughout his career, but some of his interests, such as ingestive behaviors and the effects of domestication, were not listed here.

Meyer was the most prominent figure in launching Richter's career. Just as his high school teacher had been pivotal in orienting the bright but not traditional academic to Harvard and had acted as a concerned parental guide for Richter, Meyer would also be fundamental in directing Richter's career. Who was Meyer?

ADOLF MEYER AND THE PHIPPS CLINIC AT JOHNS HOPKINS

In an obituary for the American Philosophical Society, Eliot Stellar wrote: "Curt acknowledged the debt he owed Watson even though Watson left Hopkins less than two years after Curt's arrival. It was Adolf Meyer who became the mentor and main supporter of Curt's research" (Stellar 1989). Stellar went on to acknowledge Meyer as the father of psychobiology.

A Swiss-born neurologist, Adolf Meyer studied with some of the great minds of the nineteenth century, including Hughlings Jackson. Meyer was the first head of the Phipps Psychiatric Clinic, which opened in 1913 as part of the Johns Hopkins Hospital (Harvey et al. 1989). In Meyer's view, a psychiatric clinic should include both an outpatient and an inpatient population and foster both teaching and research. The clinic's aims were to help people through both educational and therapeutic methods and to undertake laboratory research inspired by the clinic.

Before arriving at Hopkins, Meyer had held various positions in the United States, including that of clinical director of Worcester State Hospital, which was part of Clark University in Worcester, Massachusetts. Meyer was an erudite intellectual with a background and serious published works in comparative neuroanatomy. Throughout his career he taught classes in both comparative anatomy and psychobiology. Meyer emphasized whole-body activity and its long-term study and understood psychobiology as "the missing link" between "ordinary physiology and pathology . . . dealing with functions of the total person and not merely detachable parts" (Meyer 1915, p. 861).

Meyer also understood psychobiology "that takes life as it is without splitting it into something mental and something physical" (Meyer 1935, p. 94). This assertion is reminiscent of the position of James, as well as that of other pragmatists including Dewey and Mead (J. E. Smith 1978), and is very much in contrast with Watson and other behaviorists who had come to dominate psychology by this time. In other words, Meyer's psychobiology reflected an interest in "organismal function and behavior" (Meyer 1935, p. 94).

At the beginning stages of planning for the Phipps Clinic (generously endowed by Henry Phipps), the design for the Psychological Laboratory was set in motion by the selection of Watson as its head. Watson prided himself on an expertise with laboratory construction that dated back to his Chicago experience, and he was fairly involved from the start of the project, even with the electrical wiring of his own laboratory.

Once installed in his new post, Watson—behaviorism's celebrated ideologue—was overzealous in his intellectual stance that all behavior was subject to modification. Meyer became critical of Watson, although this criticism went both ways (Leys 1984; Leys and Evans 1990). Meyer was interested in functional psychobiological adaptation, not ideological dogmatism. The psychobiology he envisioned did not dismiss the inward turn of Freud or Wundt (see, for example, his correspondence with Titchener in Leys and Evans 1990), but helped to put it in perspective.

Watson and Meyer, as Leys (1984) points out, were on a collision course. Watson was having an extramarital affair with his young associate, a brash act for which he would be fired from Hopkins. Meyer apparently had an interesting stance with regard to Watson; on the one hand he seemed to support him intellectually, and on the other hand he was dead set against retaining Watson (Leys 1984; Buckley 1989). Edward Titchener, no friend to behaviorism, nevertheless berated Meyer (Leys and Evans 1990) for not supporting Watson. What Meyer cared about was a broad palette on which to paint psychology; several approaches coexisted, and perhaps most important were the adaptive regulatory responses and adjustments that had to be made for viable long-term health. Meyer's motives for not defending Watson no doubt in part reflected his distaste for the narrowness of the study of behavior that Watson paraded as the only scientific approach within psychology.

With the loss of Watson, Meyer was looking for a new head of the Psychological Laboratory. Yerkes, one of Richter's key teachers at Harvard, applied for the position, but Meyer turned him down (Buckley 1989). Instead, Meyer passed the reins to Curt Richter, who was already working independently in the laboratory, ostensibly under the guidance of Watson. Richter was somebody safe, somebody Meyer probably thought he could influence and control, somebody who would not challenge his perspective, and somebody who could set up the laboratory. In a letter, Meyer told Watson that "Yerkes offered himself as a helping hand." A little later in the same letter, he wrote, "I trust Richter will make safer contact" (Chesney Archives, April 12, 1921).

Meyer promoted a cultural context in which patients were studied over a long period. Long-term activity charts were kept on patients and included information about hygienic medicine and real-life adaptation. Meyer was a whole-body physiologist, classically trained in neurology, who had a vision of psychiatry as the treatment of the person. Perhaps Meyer's recognition of Richter's similar orientation led him to turn the key to Watson's laboratory over to Richter. Meyer did this despite the fact that Richter lacked any substantial publications and despite the fact that Watson was nominally Richter's advisor and had told him that generating good research would be enough. The laboratory was renamed the Psychobiology Laboratory.

RICHTER'S REFLECTIONS ON MEYER

In a talk titled "Reminiscences," which Curt Richter gave to Hopkins residents in the 1973/74 academic year, he described the richness of the world that Meyer created at Hopkins and how great a benefactor he was (Richter files, Chesney Archives). Richter says of Meyer, "He was always very friendly, supported all my research generously; as far as I remember he never refused a request for anything that I wanted to do. I saw a great deal of him. He popped in the lab at almost any time of the day." This relationship continued over a very important period of Richter's career, the first twenty years.

Richter was surprised to learn that Meyer helped introduce the domestic rat to the United States as a suitable laboratory animal. Richter further noted that "until about 20 years ago I hadn't really understood Dr. Meyer's enthusiastic support of my laboratory." Of course, Richter championed the rat as an ideal laboratory animal. Although Meyer did not mention Richter's work in his reviews, Richter was essential for Meyer's view of research because he represented the study of cyclical behaviors, long-term total self-regulation, and broad-based behavioral understanding.

Richter's gratitude to Meyer was expressed in a 1937 festschrift at the Phipps Clinic celebrating Meyer's seventieth birthday and his twenty-fifth year as director of the clinic. Richter said, "The place of my laboratory in the working organization of the Phipps is difficult to describe along orthodox lines. As I look back over its development I am sure it could never have flourished anywhere else except under Dr. Meyer's broad and tolerant point of view and aided by his guidance, encouragement and constructive criticism" (Richter 1938e, p. 81).

In his early years, Richter reached out to Meyer, and Meyer reciprocated as a scientific parent might; it is clear that Richter saw him as a father figure. In letters to Meyer, Richter asked for counsel and support and told Meyer about his trips and about what equipment and funds he needed.

Clearly, Richter looked to Meyer as his confidante, for intellectual guidance, and for practical advice and help. He saw Meyer as an all-purpose, friendly figure who had Richter's interests at heart. And those interests furthered the development of the Phipps Clinic as a place for the patient, a place to be educated, and a place for research.

The Phipps Psychiatric Clinic was Meyer's baby, his home, and Richter described Meyer as "at heart a Swiss hotel-keeper. Everything in the Phipps had to be watched over carefully as a good Swiss hotel-manager would do" (Richter files, Chesney Archives, 1974). Richter was the fortunate benefactor in every possible way, and Meyer set the stage by putting Richter in position as head of the laboratory and supporting him through the first twenty years of his long career.

In some of their correspondence during this early period, there is clearly some tension between Richter and Meyer (in part having to do with Richter's divorce). The young Curt Richter also felt some pressure from his dependent relationship with Meyer, his chief. In a letter from Richter to Meyer dated August 26, 1929, he stated:

> I am writing to tell you what I would like to do next year and to offer a concrete
> plan which I hope will serve the purpose of helping us to arrive at a constructive
> working agreement and thereby bring to a close what has been for me a very

unhappy period. I am glad to state at once that I should like to withdraw my res-
ignation and assume all of my old responsibilities along with others concerned
with the working out of the course in psychobiology. The latter responsibility I
assume willingly and gladly since during the summer my resistance to giving a
course of this kind has largely disappeared. I feel that now I can undertake this
work with confidence as well as with enthusiasm. I may also state at once that I
will give you my word that I will take care of the settlement of marital difficulties
and the associated complications in a way that is in harmony with your own personal wishes and the interests of the Phipps clinic. (Meyer files, Chesney
Archives)

Richter wanted to mend fences with Meyer, to let Meyer know that he was
eager to teach the course, and to put his "difficulties" (issues about his marriage) behind him. Meyer controlled Richter from a power position. Meyer, the
"Swiss innkeeper" of the Phipps, wanted neither scientific nor personal scan-
dal. Hopkins had a history of removing individuals for having extramarital
affairs (e.g., Peirce, Baldwin, Watson). In fact, Meyer would ask prospective
faculty, "Do you consider marriage as a contract binding for life at all possible? . . . Would you consider yourself justified to intrude between married
people: in other words what is your attitude towards adultery and flirtation
with married persons?" (Meyer files, Chesney Archives).

Meyer, perhaps having had enough of Watson's partying and rough ways,
sought safety and calm and was puritanical in orientation. Richter was safe
because he needed Meyer and was under his control. Later he remembered
Meyer with affection and gratitude.

When asked about his experience with Meyer, Richter said that he had "all
the opportunities I could ask for." When asked about how much he had had to
do with the psychiatric patients, he said, "During Dr. Meyer's time, I spent a
lot of time in the clinic. After Dr. Whitethorn came in, a real change took place
in Phipps. . . . The patients were turned over to individual doctors—they no
longer were seen by everyone" (Roe, second interview, American Philosophical
Society Archives, 1962). He went on to describe the high degree of interaction
he had had with patients when Meyer was chief. These were important experiences because they exposed Richter to clinical issues. During Word War II
Richter kept doing clinical work with galvanic skin measurement and assess-
ment of brain damage (see chapter 5), but his integration into the culture of the
Phipps as a daily affair changed with the departure of Meyer.

Richter, in a presentation and subsequent publication entitled "A Biological Approach to Manic Depressive Insanity," noted that "a person who has well-organized habits of work, a wide range of interests, and accessible outlets, would be able to take care of the excess of energy in a well-organized way. Such a person was Roosevelt" (Richter 1930a). Meyer, commenting on Richter's paper, asserted that "we are dealing with a number of systems, and not one unitary system underlying the activity/inactivity; this is the work that stems from Richter's thesis. The total organism in adaptation to its surroundings is under study" (Richter 1930a, pp. 621–22).

Meyer set the rich and varied intellectual context for the clinic. A close reading of *The Collected Papers of Adolf Meyer* (1951) reveals great intellectual acumen—he was so well read, so much the European intellectual in the United States. But he was in the United States, and though Hopkins was modeled on German research institutions, the United States was less constrained by the straitjacket of tradition. Richter noted in an unpublished essay that Meyer went on a boat trip to Boston from Baltimore "chiefly to hear a lecture by William James. That was really the high point of his life" (Richter files, Chesney Archives). The influence of the legacy of this American classical pragmatist on Meyer was apparent to Richter.

MEYER, RICHTER, AND AMERICAN PRAGMATISM

While he was at Worcester, Meyer had interacted with James, who, along with C. S. Peirce and John Dewey, had influenced him. He liked what he called their "instrumentalism." Indeed, Meyer was impressed with his new country and its sense of pragmatism. "It was the work of American thinkers, especially of Charles S. Peirce, of John Dewey and of William James, which justified in us a basic sense of pluralism, that is to say, a recognition that nature is not just one smooth continuity" (Meyer 1951, 2:28; see also Leys 1984; Leys and Evans 1990). It was in American pragmatism and its biological adaptation, problem solving, and whole-body activity (Schneider 1946/1963), that Meyer located psychobiology (Klerman 1979).

Meyer's interest in "organismal total function," was passed on to Richter, and he found a compatible philosophical approach in American pragmatism and his new country. Meyer no doubt saw in Richter a shared piece of the Old World from which he had emigrated and the expression of the German language, but also the newfound freedom, the "roll-up-your-sleeves" pluralism of the country in which he now found himself. Perhaps Meyer looked at the young

Richter and saw the outward expression of this point of view. As Meyer put it, "The factors at work in the development of a psychobiological conception had much support in American thought. Pluralism and pragmatism were liberating factors in throwing off dogmatic dualism" (Meyer 1931/1957, p. 47). A little later in the same paragraph, he described "William James' clear vision of the significance of the pragmatism of Charles S. Peirce and the instrumentalism of John Dewey, and the healthy encouragement given to natural spontaneity of thought and work in the American environment" (Meyer 1931/1957, p. 47).

Invention and experimentation predominate in a pragmatic orientation. Pragmatism is a philosophy of experimentalism (Dewey 1916) and represents "the open air and possibilities of nature" (James 1907/1958, p. 45). This open sensibility was an important theme in many of the pragmatists' conceptions (Dewey 1925/1989) and is consistent with what Richter called "free research" (Richter 1953f). Free research is close to open-ended, unencumbered inquiry, something dear to the pragmatists and certainly to Richter.

C. S. Peirce can be credited with creating the first psychology laboratory in the United States, which he did at Johns Hopkins in the 1870s (Cadwallader 1974). The laboratory spirit of Peirce and his pragmatism (1877, 1898/1992) meant that the universe could be opened through experiment (J. E. Smith 1978). Scientific inquiry was rough and ready, biologically grounded in human and animal problem solving. A persistent feature of this orientation, at least for James, was that "pragmatism is uncomfortable away from facts" (James 1907/1958, p. 54). Richter was also uncomfortable away from experiments and the facts derived from experiments.

Meyer oriented his psychobiological perspective to that of American pragmatism. One inquirer put it this way: "I had long been puzzled—since I first met Adolf Meyer and recognized the similarity of his teachings to those of James and Dewey—how it happened that a Swiss had embraced pragmatism, indeed had found in it his natural voice" (Lidz 1966, p. 323; see also Leys 1984). In the cultural air breathed by Richter and his immediate predecessors, evolution and Darwin figured prominently. The great *Principles of Psychology* (James 1890/1952) was rich in biological perspective, functional utility, and evolutionary conceptions. Dewey had no less of an influence, and one of his early works, at the turn of the twentieth century, was *The Influence of Darwin on Philosophy* (Dewey 1910/1965). Dewey received his degree at Hopkins and was one of its first graduate students. Knowledge acquisition was now linked to adaptation; the intellectual generation immediately before Richter had struggled to incorporate the new insights of Darwin into current thinking. These insights swept across Europe and reached the United States. By the end of the nineteenth and early twentieth centuries, the cultural milieu was ripe for the acceptance of the first biological revolution, a conception of biological adaptation. Richter inherited a pragmatism that was tied to the version of nineteenth-century biological thinking that permeated Harvard and later Hopkins through Meyer. These concepts were perhaps implicit for an engineer bent on exploring the biological basis of behavior, and Richter relied on this sense of pragmatism to discern how things worked. Richter never doubted the validity of the scientific method.

THE ROE INTERVIEW

In 1949, the psychologist Anne Roe contacted Richter for her 1953 book *The Making of a Scientist.* Roe, a Ph.D. psychologist and the wife of the noted evolutionary biologist George Gaylord Simpson, interviewed scientists for the book. Roe had received a grant to look at the "personalities of scientists in different fields" (November 22, 1949) and to determine their "life history." The psychologists she interviewed included Karl Lashley, B. F. Skinner, Donald Lindsey, Stanley Smith Stevens, Jerome Bruner, and Ernest Hilgard. Roe approached Richter about being a subject, and he replied, "You may count me as a guinea pig" (letter to Roe, American Philosophical Society Archives, December 1949).

The interviewees were questioned extensively about their life histories and were given Rorschach tests. In her summary statement (American Philosophical Society Archives, March 1952), Roe referred to Richter as "always a poor student in any sort of formal instruction . . . who thinks, I am sure correctly, that under the present set-up he would never have gotten anywhere." A little later she wrote, "The only argument [is] whether or not he was a psychologist rather than a zoologist or something else." She also noted that "[Richter] himself feels his closest professional contacts are not with *psychologists,* although it was they who put him in the National Academy."

Richter and Roe's relationship would be long-lasting, and from their correspondence it is evident that they were friendly with each other. Both Roe and her husband, like Richter, had grown up in Denver, and in some of their discussions they reminisced about the old days in that city. Roe noted in her summary that she had actually met Richter in 1924 in Denver.

Roe commented about Richter's life, his parents, his two marriages ("his present wife, obviously a southerner") and his children (he had three, two with his first wife and one with his second), his athletic prowess, the importance of his high school teacher, his authoritarian father, his German background and experiences, his love of free play and the permissiveness of his mother in letting him engage in just that, his experiences at Harvard and in the army, his arrival at Hopkins and his relationship with Watson, and, of course, the importance of Meyer to the development of his scientific sensibility and the origins of his scientific career. In fact, Richter said of Meyer that he was "the greatest scholar I had ever come into contact with. He had a great fund of information and high ideals of tolerance" (Roe interviews, American Philosophical Society Archives, March 1952).

Roe also wrote about the results of Rorschach tests of Richter, which indicated that he was detached, not particularly orderly, a bit stubborn, and "conventional but not impulsive about it." Of course, she would realize just how much he could reach out, because they would have a long-term relationship. The interview would continue after Roe received a grant from the National Institute of Mental Health to look at changes in the scientists since the first series of interviews. She wrote to Richter on October 1, 1962, and said "no tests" this time. She wanted to know about the productivity of the scientists in the ensuing years. When she asked, "Are you still working full-time?" he responded, "Oh sure, I'm emeritus for three years now, and they are letting me stay on for five, possibly ten years." In fact, he would stay much longer than that. In this interview, he mentioned his doctoral thesis and his recent trip to Princeton, where he had spent a year. Roe asked him questions about graduate students, and he suggested that many of them did not work very hard and that money was being wasted on them (letter to Roe, American Philosophical Society Archives).

Richter wrote to Roe, "This is to tell you how much I enjoyed your visit" (November 20, 1962). In a letter dated June 16, 1970, he told her, "It was such fun to see you and George again. I regretted so much that we couldn't have more time together."

The information on Richter in the Roe interviews was quite consistent with his autobiography. Anne Roe also sent him a copy of what she wrote about him, and he obviously felt comfortable with it. Their letters included many references back to Denver, the local high school, and their earlier years. Richter enjoyed his connection to Roe's husband, George Gaylord Simpson, one of the leading evolutionary biologists of his time. They met on occasion at the American Philosophical Society in Philadelphia, to which Simpson was elected in 1936 and Richter in 1959.

THE AMERICAN PHILOSOPHICAL SOCIETY: THE STUDY OF PRACTICAL PHILOSOPHY

C. S. Peirce, the preeminent pragmatist, defined the meaning of a concept by its broadly conceived practical consequences (Peirce 1878). Founded in the eighteenth century, the American Philosophical Society, with its emphasis on the practical implications of discovery, was a forerunner of this American pragmatism. The society was the first American intellectual society and was devoted to "promoting useful knowledge." Its orientation was toward invention. Richter surely was at home in this world.

A sense of experimentalism has always run through American inquiry. The work and thought of Jonathan Edwards, Benjamin Franklin, and Thomas Jefferson are just a few examples. Inventions and methodological innovations have always been part and parcel of epistemological advances (Schneider 1946/1963; J. E. Smith 1978). Curt Richter, too, was grounded in invention and experimentation.

By all accounts, Richter enjoyed his membership in the society, which was founded by Benjamin Franklin, its first president; its third president was Thomas Jefferson. The legacy of Franklin, a precursor to what would become American pragmatism, surely was a comfortable fit for Richter. Inquiry was the dominant mode—a laboratory state of mind.

With selected individuals, Richter carved out a rich social life. By all accounts, he enjoyed the aristocratic role of the gentleman scientist, a class of individual belonging to the "right" social clubs. For Richter, those clubs included the American Philosophical Society, the National Academy of Sciences, and the Hamilton Street Club (an elite social club in Baltimore), which provided him with colleagues and social status.

Richter maintained a long relationship with the psychologist Leonard Carmichel, a physiological psychologist (whose students included Carl Pfaffmann) who would become the president of the American Philosophical Society and the secretary of the Smithsonian Institution. Richter was on familiar terms with Simon Flexner, the leader and one of the founders of the Rockefeller Institute and one of the founders of the Institute for Advanced Studies at Princeton. Richter lived in a rarified world of science. He warranted it, and he had the good fortune to experience it.

RICHTER'S APPROACH TO RESEARCH

Richter was never oriented toward experimental design or statistical analysis. He was always oriented to measurement, to biological adaptation and the engineering design of animal biology, and to the recognition of individual differences. He said of himself that he thought in terms of instruments. With his colleagues, he emphasized the evidence of rhythms (J. Wirth and T. Moran, pers. comm., August 2002), rather than debating the concept of biological rhythms itself. Richter always had a nose for what to investigate.

Richter was intellectually close to Claude Bernard, who enunciated a philosophy of experimentation and of applying the method of simple experimentation to the study of physiological regulation (Holmes 1974, 2004). Bernard noted that a "created organism is a machine which necessarily works by virtue of the physico-chemical properties of its constitute elements" (1865/1957, p. 93). Richter took this to heart and extended it to organismic biology. What Richter did not embrace was the logic of statistical design and probabilities. There was little of statistical prowess in Richter's concept of experimentation. He worked with a relatively small number of subjects and followed them over a long period. Richter invented machinery for measurement and was a surgical genius.

Richter explored phenomena, and, remarkably, he stayed interested in several core research focuses over his career of more than sixty years. He developed some research tools that he used for the duration of his career, but he would continue to expand the range of his surgical skill. Richter often thought with his hands, with his laboratory construction, or with his surgical innovations.

His style of research was innovative, artful, esthetic, and playful. And he was always anchored to a sense of behavioral adaptation. He described himself as "scavenger-like" in his approach to science, using the resources that were available, expanding the tools for research.

CONCLUSION

Richter entered a rich intellectual milieu in which the culture of research was prominent. He was less comfortable in the world of ideas than in the world of instruments. He let others take their positions while he remained steadfast to what he discovered in his laboratory. Of course, he presupposed some ideas critical to his research. He did not take it as his task to argue for his ideas. He was fortunate; the ideas that he inhabited and inherited were rich, and his ingenuity and scientific fearlessness (in the sense that he was unafraid to explore a wide variety of biological phenomena) were quite extraordinary. He was lucky that he emerged when he did.

Coming to Hopkins in the second decade of the twentieth century, Richter was in the perfect place for a career in the nascent field of behavioral biology, or psychobiology; the Phipps Clinic was a unique setting for a unique investigator (McHugh 1989). Richter was a craftsman and, as such, was comfortable in the laboratory. Richter was also an inventor who was temperamentally close to functional explanations. Richter's sense of adventure and his effort, two key themes of his life and work, paralleled the pragmatic thread throughout his career.

In his autobiography, Richter characterized himself as having had his research gene released. This is a striking metaphor, revelatory of his concept of himself and the nature of his studies. Innate structure, genetically endowed, was the formidable intellectual concept that guided almost all of Richter's research.

Adolf Meyer set the stage for Curt Richter; the link to pragmatism and broadly conceived behavioral adaptation and self-regulation became an important part of Richter's scientific investigations. Meyer must have seen in Richter the great scientist that he would become, the artisan laboratory inventor and experimentalist.

Curt Richter has been called the "compleat psychobiologist" (Rozin 1976a) for his scientific ingenuity, artistry, and discovery. As Rozin put it, "Richter truly deserves the title, the compleat psychobiologist. . . . for the range and richness of his approach" (Rozin 1976a, p. xvii). His scientific range encompassed the fields of psychobiology, behavioral endocrinology, and behavioral medicine. His discoveries included the regulation of spontaneous behaviors, homeostatic and nutrition selection, wild and domesticated rat expression, and neurological discovery and invention.

Richter inhabited a world of ideas not to be engaged theoretically, but to be demonstrated in the laboratory. It was the laboratory demonstration that captured Richter's imagination, the challenge of generating new instruments and inventing new ways to measure behavior. Curt Richter, oriented as an engineer to build artifacts of ingenuity, found his niche as an experimentalist. The field was new, and the time was ripe to begin a scientific harvest that still yields results today.

CHAPTER 2

Biological Clocks and Spontaneous Behaviors

Curt Richter commented on his own youthful tinkering that he "spent a lot of time working on locks and clocks—taking them apart and putting them back together again" (Richter 1985, p. 359). Richter began his research career by studying cyclic behavior and what many called "spontaneous behaviors." Richter's career began with the clocks and ended with the clocks. They were his first scientific love and a lasting romance.

A romantic vision of nature coupled with an engineering perspective on design and adaptation permeated Richter's work on biological clocks and their role in regulatory physiology. Moreover, he saw behavior not as an appendage or aberration, but as an essential ingredient of physiological regulation. Clocks help generate the behaviors animals use to perform activities vital for their survival. Clocks, in Richter's view, are not subject to external perturbation, but trigger a variety of adaptive behaviors—an engineering principle that allows behavioral flexibility and problem solving.

Richter understood biological clocks as fundamental to the organization of behavior and physiological adaptation. In fact, before Richter there were limited experimental contexts for inquiry into biological clocks and their role in the regulation of behavior, though there had been some discussion of them, notably by Johnson (1926). The role of clocks in regulating behavior and physiology, particularly in mammals, would not be fully understood for decades (Rusak and Zucker 1979; Rosenwasser and Adler 1986).

PSYCHOLOGY AS SCIENCE

The field of psychology was new and searching for legitimacy when Richter first encountered it. It had links to two different historical traditions: (1) the rationalism of Descartes (and modern rationalism), and (2) Hume and modern empiricism. Kant and other forerunners of modern cognitive science tried to synthesize the two traditions. Before the search for the legitimacy of knowledge became embedded in modern epistemology, there was the sound, commonsense psychology of Aristotle and other classical writers about the human condition and its wants and desires.

The intellectual climate in which Richter found himself at the start of his career was rooted in the work of Darwin and William James. The influence of Darwinism was enormous. Despite the rejection of Darwin by James's biology professor, Louis Agassiz, at Harvard, (S. J. Gould 2002), William James embraced the biological perspective that was revolutionizing the sciences, and he incorporated this perspective into his conception of psychology. *The Principles of Psychology* (James 1890/1952) remains one of the most important books in psychology; few textbooks have had such lasting allure. James's pragmatism was fused to his functionalism: What were the functions of a set of behaviors? For James, psychological events were to be understood partly within the context of biological adaptation (James 1890/1952). The same approach would pervade Richter's work.

The goal of the science of psychology, however, was the continued realization of science—positive knowledge. Recall that during this period university philosophy and psychology departments were not separate. Psychology, as James understood it, was the study of the mind. But, again, the mind was not something ethereal; it was functional. For James, the subcomponents of the machinery of the mind, such as attention, were linked to the degree of information that could be processed (James 1890/1952). The emotions, for James and Darwin, evolved as aids to problem solving, which was the basis of functional psychology and was biologically based (Darwin 1872/1998).

One dominant issue for those thinking about the study of behavior was what constituted a real science of psychology. The so-called Subjective school (Titchener 1929/1972) concerned itself primarily with introspection. The issue of introspection was suspect and forbidden for Watson. "Objectivism," as behaviorism was sometimes called early on, was simply an approach to measuring behavior. During its early years, the stakes for psychology were high, consisting of no less than legitimacy in the scientific community.

Both during Richter's time and earlier, several already legitimate systems competed for expression in physiological neurobiology, which was anchored to psychological functions (Broca 1861/1960). These included clinical teachings linked to the study of drives (Freud 1920/1975) and a formidable tradition in the field of psychophysics (Fechner 1860/1966; Helmholtz 1867/1963; Boring 1929/1950; Hilgard 1987). Adolf Meyer, who had been educated in these ideas in Europe, transmitted the rich continental tradition to the young Richter.

Closer to home at Hopkins, and elsewhere, were the great debates between vitalism and tropism (Jennings 1907; Loeb 1918/1973). These debates centered on the question of what were the underlying experimental and conceptual frameworks for behavior and psychology (Pauly 1987). Richter was intrigued by many intellectual disciplines, but he did not belong to any of them in any real sense, at least not at the level of public debate of ideas.

The battle was on for how to make psychology into science. Robert Yerkes (1903, 1913), well known for his comparative work, set out to study the biological basis of behavior and, in particular, comparative intelligence. Yerkes interacted with many competing voices, including Watson's, but Yerkes came out finally for the study of "organic behavior." Psychobiology, for Yerkes, as it would be for Richter, was about biological adaptation (Yerkes 1921, 1930).

PSYCHOBIOLOGY

When Richter set up his laboratory, a few individuals had written on the subject of psychobiology. These included Knight Dunlap, a psychologist at Hopkins. Dunlap's book on psychobiology made some reference to behavior, but very little (Dunlap 1914); further discovery would await Richter (see Dewsbury 1991 for a history of psychobiology). Meyer, like many other investigators of the day, provided his own orientation to the study of psychobiology. The emphasis for Meyer was on "total self-regulatory behavior." This would be a constant experimental theme for Richter. Indeed, Richter went far beyond Meyer, who remained wholly theoretical. In contrast to Meyer, Richter rarely looked up from his data.

There are a number of meanings associated with the term *psychobiology* (Dewsbury 1991). Perhaps the clearest sense is that which posits biological explanations for behavior. Meyer, who wrote extensively on this topic, emphasized long-term adaptation and organismic responses to ecological perturbations (see also Dewey 1925/1989).

PSYCHOBIOLOGY AND CLOCKS

Richter thought cyclic behaviors were internally generated. Two issues stood out for him: regularity and uniformity. These would be themes in all of his work on biological rhythms, as would the idea that pathology revealed important sources of information about the normal function of the clocks.

Clocks keep time and provide the order and coherence required by the outer world to which we try to adapt. Cyclical representations have a long history, which Richter appreciated. Harmonic relationships, as Greek thinkers understood, represent the cycles of events. Many thinkers over the years embraced the cyclic nature of events and their fixed patterns of expression. With the advent of Darwinism, fitness and long-term survival became linked to cyclical events. The study of the clocks that underlie behavior anchored research to real-world events and to a prized human invention, the mechanical objects made for measuring and depicting time.

The biological revolution was at hand: Darwin's revelations about adaptation, speciation, secondary sexual characteristics, and problem solving. The machinery varied in design and niche because nature selected the features of good fit.

Richter embraced two key questions. The first involved the idea of machine design: How would an engineer design a particular behavioral or physiological expression? The second was: What were the causes of spontaneous expression? These themes reflected the horns of the dilemma of determinism versus free expression.

INTERNALLY GENERATED BEHAVIORS: A VIEW OF SPONTANEOUS BEHAVIORS

Bernard noted that "spontaneity enjoyed by beings endowed with life has been one of the objections urged against the use of experimentation in biological studies" (Bernard 1865/1957, p. 5). Richter believed that spontaneous expression was an outgrowth of biological clocks. This would constitute, in part, a solution to the problem of spontaneous behaviors.

In Richter's view, the clocks themselves were fixed. Spontaneous behaviors were a way to conceive of animal behavior that was internally generated and not externally caused. Of course, the clocks reflected the events of nature, the daily and seasonal rhythms. The internal generators were at the heart of spontaneous behavior; they were biologically based. Again, one has to place this in a historical setting, namely, Watson's laboratory (Rozin 1976a). Moreover, the generators were something that an engineer could understand. For example, an engineer could design a piece of machinery to express something every twelve hours on the clock despite rain or snow. Spontaneous behavior reflected internal generators under the mechanism of natural selection, serving a behaviorally and physiologically adaptive set of functions. Thus, biological cycles were internally generated.

In his first major review, "A Behavioristic Study of the Activity of the Rat," Richter laid out his approach to the study of behavior (Richter 1922). But this bore no resemblance to the behaviorism of Watson. Again, what Richter meant by a "behavioristic" study was the measurement of behavior, something objective. Behavior, Richter (echoing Meyer) argued, was about the whole organism adapting to circumstances. "Interest in human psychology is moving rapidly toward problems of general adaptation involving responses of the whole organism in actual working life situations" (Richter 1922, p. 1).

Richter outlined an approach in which the various organ systems of the individual would be studied, not in isolation from one another, but as a "total organism." For purposes of objectivity, he would first derive measures of an animal's activities—eating, drinking, moving, defecating, and other activities—under ordinary conditions, and then look at these behaviors under irregular conditions or perturbations. Richter wanted to understand what he called "the dynamic of behavior" or, quoting Meyer, "experiments of nature"—diseases of normal behavioral expression. After all, Richter worked in a psychiatric clinic where curing behavior was a fundamental end point of inquiry. But Richter's approach was as an engineer in a clinical setting. He was concerned with determining the origins and mechanisms of animal activity.

THE STUDY OF SPONTANEOUS BEHAVIOR

Before Richter there was a paucity of research investigation on animal activity. Richter would create a way to measure behavior and what he called the study of "gross bodily activity" by developing an activity cage and manipulating variables such as light.

Richter monitored the whole activity of the animal with his multiple-cage activity method (fig. 2.1). He suggested that the multiple-cage approach would produce an animal more "intelligent," or more fit, than those raised in less enriched environments (Richter 1922, 1927a). Other researchers would eventually show that enriched environments could foster cortical changes and facilitate a broad array of problem-solving proclivities not seen in rats raised in more impoverished environments (e.g., Rosenzweig and Bennett 1996).

In his thesis Richter developed numerous ways to monitor behavior. For the activity cage, for example, Richter attached to the corner of each cage a

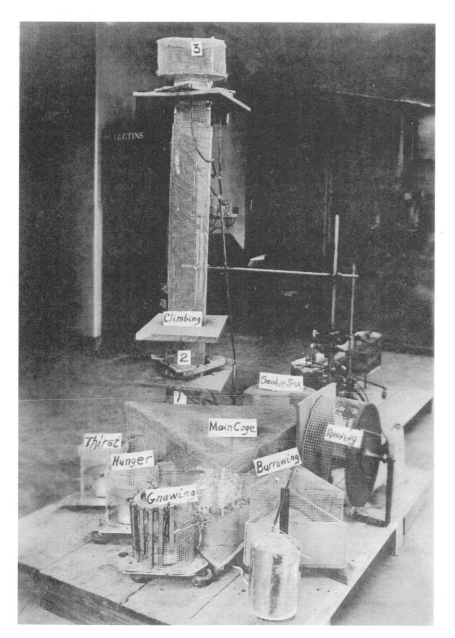

FIG. 2.1. Activity chambers in which various behaviors were monitored, including thirst, hunger, gnawing, running, burrowing, climbing, and mating. *Source:* Richter 1927a

"rubber membrane tightly over a large tambour. The tambours are connected together immediately under the cage into one tube which is led to a small Marey tambour, the lever of which records on the smoked paper of a kymograph." Every movement of an animal, even the slightest, was recorded on the drum with a single mark (Richter 1922, p. 5).

In his experiments, Richter observed alternating patterns of activity and inactivity in rats. He noted that the patterns of active behavior varied between individual rats and with age. In young rats, the rate of alternation between activity and inactivity was much greater than in older animals. Richter noted that this pattern of behavioral alternation was present in the newborn rat and presumably was an innate, hard-wired behavioral pattern expressed in a variety of animal species.

Richter then asked, what happens to the activity patterns when external conditions vary? Say, with hunger? Rats were given a diet adapted from McCollum, a nutritionist at Hopkins. (Many of Richter's diets were derived from the McCollum diets; see chapter 3.) He noted that activity initially increased when the animals were deprived of food but given access to water but began to decline by the fourth day without food. By contrast, rats deprived of both water and food had decreased activity levels very early in the experiments.

Richter showed that rats were inactive after a bout of eating. This phenomenon would later be linked to "postprandial satiety," in which inactivity after a meal is indicative of the mechanisms of digestion and absorption. G. Smith would later comment that one of the figures from Richter's 1922 paper "depicted the critical part of the satiety sequence. . . . When rats stop eating, they engage in a brief period of non-feeding activity before they rest and go to sleep" (G. P. Smith, 1989, p. 1).

Richter's next step in varying environmental factors and meals was to look at how single meals interacted with activity and drinking patterns and how constant light or different temperatures affected the expression of activity or inactivity. Long periods of darkness, high temperatures, and low temperatures influenced activity patterns. He noted the changes in expression of the activity/inactivity distribution.

Richter noted that rats are nocturnal; they were more active when the lights were off than when they were on. Richter also observed that rats became more nocturnal with increasing age. His work demonstrated that hunger, light, and temperature all altered spontaneous behaviors.

Richter and his colleagues at both the Phipps Clinic and Columbia University observed the sleep patterns of human infants and the alternating expression of activity and inactivity (Richter 1922; Wada 1922). They learned that the origins of gross bodily activity or spontaneous activity are independent of external stimuli. For further research, it would be important to find a way to distinguish and measure levels of activity and the cyclicity of activity.

Richter's thesis work was a breakthrough in the laboratory study of behavior. From his monitoring of eating and drinking and other activity patterns, one could gain a real idea of the behavior of the rat and the effects of manipulations such as food deprivation and alteration of light/dark cycles on that behavior. This orientation toward behavioral analysis would set the tone for the rest of his career.

STOMACH CONTRACTIONS AND ACTIVITY: A PERIPHERALIST PERSPECTIVE

Richter investigated different organ systems and, under the influence of Carlson (1916) and Cannon (1915/1929), focused on the contractions of the stomach, which were thought to be linked to food appetite and activity. Richter hypothesized that the endogenous contractions of the stomach might influence gross activity and inactivity. His results suggested that when the stomach was quiescent, activity diminished; the converse held when the stomach contracted intensely. Contractions of the stomach, when isolated, were periodic and therefore contained an autonomous or endogenous function (Carlson 1916). Richter asserted as the principle that dominated his inquiry that "there is a tendency in all living organisms to maintain a metabolic balance or equilibrium" (Richter 1922). Richter understood as homeostatic regulation the activity and inactivity used to maintain internal balance. The stomach, Richter noted, might not be the only peripheral organ linked to activity and inactivity.

Richter mistakenly placed great weight on the contractions of the stomach, and he thought their intensity was linked to degree of hunger (Richter 1922, 1927a; Cannon 1915/1929; Carlson 1916). When food reached the stomach, Richter suggested, contractions decreased, and food activity and food ingestion decreased as well. Richter noted, however, that he was never able in his animal studies simultaneously to monitor activity, feeding, and stomach contractions (Richter 1922). Nonetheless, he held the view that rats' activity and orientation to food sources were related to stomach contractions.

This theme of internal drives and spontaneous behavior continued in Richter's 1927 paper, in which he noted that a two-hour running activity reflected gastric contractions in laboratory animals. A comparative perspective predominated as Richter looked at several species. Richter and his students and colleagues in the early 1920s observed human newborns, rats, and other species to discern the role of the stomach in animal activity, drives, and orientation toward objects. They studied the whole of animal activity. However, not a statistic can be found among their research data, which was not uncommon in Richter's day.

Richter suggested that rats eat, under his laboratory conditions, about seven times a day. Drinking was associated with eating in the laboratory, and Richter found that the rat drank about ten times a day, at intervals of about two and a half hours. Of course, this depended on the water content of the food and the link between drinking and eating (see, e.g., Kissileff and Epstein 1969). Richter again monitored the whole activity, from what went into the animal to what went out of the animal. Richter was beginning to establish an important role of internal oscillators (Richter 1922), that "the regulatory anticipation of the feeding periods may also be explained on the basis of the clock-like functioning of the internal organ" (Blass 1976, p. 43).

A decade later, in an influential article, Karl Lashley noted that the sustained motivation for food of food-deprived animals did not depend on the two-hour rhythmic patterns generated by the stomach (Lashley 1938/1960). Neural programs generated the motivation to search for food (Hebb 1949; Stellar 1954). Moreover, we now know that stomach contractions, and the stomach in general, play a role in food satiety (e.g., Wirth and McHugh 1983) but are neither necessary nor sufficient to initiate hunger (G. P. Smith 1997). Instead, the brain orchestrates the behavior. Richter was still under the spell of the peripheralist physiological perspective (e.g., Cannon 1915/1929) which was part of the zeitgeist.

ORGAN SYSTEMS THAT INFLUENCE ACTIVITY

Richter was one of the founders of behavioral endocrinology. He looked at natural variation in the endocrine cycle as well as the influence of removing endocrine tissue and of injecting hormones to replace a lost endocrine system. His approach, as always, was concrete; in many of these experiments he removed tissue from the gland in question and placed it elsewhere in the body, in some cases injecting it into the corner of the eye (Richter 1956d).

The Gonadal Organs. Richter and his colleagues studied the effects of the ovarian cycle on spontaneous behaviors. They corroborated and extended the finding that the ovarian cycle in the rat operates on a four-day activity rhythm (Wang, Richter, and Guttmacher 1925).

Wang found that running activity was at its highest during sexual receptivity in the female rat and that running, cycling, and receptivity depended on ovarian secretion or function. Removal of the ovaries reduced the running activity and ovarian grafts restored it (Wang, Richter, and Guttmacher 1925).

Richter and Hartman (1934) demonstrated that gonadectomy dramatically decreased running activity and that replacement by gonadal transplant restored activity patterns. Wang, Richter, and Guttmacher (1925) noted an important sex difference: females ran faster and longer than males. They found that running activity was less altered by removal of the testes in males than by removal of the ovaries in females and that implants of ovary extracts in males increased their running activity.

Because Richter's work was housed in a hospital, he had access to patients and medical resources. In an interesting study, he exposed gonadectomized male and female rats, via graduated drinking tubes, to the urine of women who were seven to nine months pregnant. Richter wondered whether the products in the urine would affect running activity. The result: the running activity of ovariectomized females returned to normal, and vaginal smears demonstrated a physiological effect (fig. 2.2). Richter inferred that estrogen and other substances in the urine had effects on both running activity and the reproductive tract (Richter 1934d).

The Pituitary Gland. Hypophysectomy decreased spontaneous running activity in rats (Richter and Eckert 1936). Injections of various pituitary extracts restored the activity. Again, as in all experiments, Richter and his colleagues provided means of animals over days. Changes in end-organ systems were noted; there were decreases in the size of the thyroid, gonadal, adrenal, and pancreatic glands. Replacement therapy, both by injection and by implanting tissue on the corner of the eye, restored to various degrees the behavioral and physiological functions of these end organ systems.

The Adrenal Gland. Adrenalectomy dramatically decreased running activity and adrenal implants restored it (Richter 1936c). Richter surmised that the cortical tissue facilitated recovery, and indeed this is where aldosterone—the salt-retaining hormone—is synthesized. Richter noted that the survival rate

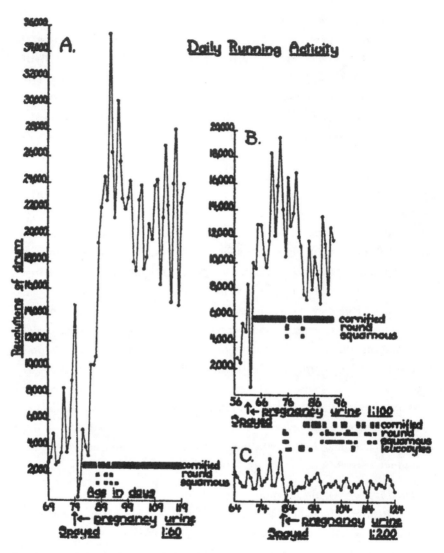

FIG. 2.2. A: The effect of pregnancy urine in 1:60 dilution on the daily running activity of a spayed female rat; also the effect on the reproductive tract manifested in the vaginal smears. B: The effect of pregnancy urine in 1:100 dilution on activity and the reproductive tract. C: The effect of pregnancy urine in 1:200 dilution on activity and the reproductive tract. *Source:* Richter 1934d

after adrenalectomy was less than 50 percent. He inferred that two hormones in the adrenal gland were essential; one kept the animal alive and the other kept it running.

By changing its glandular function and competence through adrenalectomy Richter challenged a rat's internal milieu, its metabolic and nutrient balance (see chapter 3). But in several experiments, he directly manipulated diet to determine the effects on running activity.

The Thyroid and Parathyroid Glands. Thyroidectomy also decreased running activity in rats. Richter had already noted this variation in behavioral activity and the important endocrine characteristic that just a small amount of endocrine tissue was necessary for running activity to be expressed to its full extent. This would become an important theme in the ablation studies and the behavioral performance of many end-organ systems. The replacement of thyroid extracts restored running activity in thyroidectomized rats, and their water and food intake returned to normal (Richter 1933c).

Richter noted that thyroid levels affected biological rhythmic behaviors. The reduction of thyroid hormone levels routinely decreased activity. Moreover, parathyroidectomy, which affected calcium metabolism (see chapter 3), also affected rhythmic behavior (Richter 1933c). Both endocrine systems were subsequently linked to behavioral activation and depressive states in humans (McEachron and Schull 1993). Ablation of the thyroid gland rendered the rat vulnerable to thermal dysregulation, the behavioral adaptation for which was nest building. The behaviors all increased heat production, through running.

BEHAVIORAL REGULATION OF TEMPERATURE

Richter's dissertation included work on the nest-building activities of the rat. He continued this work with Elaine Kinder, who did the research for her Ph.D. in Richter's laboratory and further demonstrated the elaborate nest-building behaviors of the laboratory rat (Kinder 1927), measuring the number of paper strips rats used to build their nests (fig. 2.3).

Once again, Richter argued that the expression of nest building is "practically independent of experience, since young rats 30 days old raised in sawdust build a perfect nest out of the crepe paper the first time it is presented to them" (Richter 1927a, p. 88; Blass 1976). These behavioral responses are instinctual or innate. Richter demonstrated in the laboratory an important

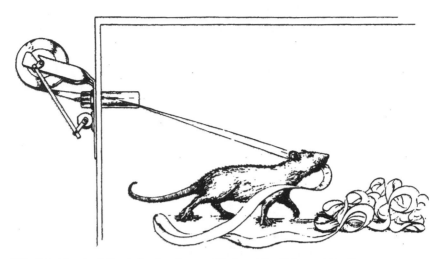

FIG. 2.3. Nest-building behavior. *Source:* Kinder 1927; Richter 1942–43

behavioral adaptation in the regulation of the internal milieu, namely, the behavioral regulation of temperature homeostasis.

THE CIRCADIAN CLOCK

One key feature that facilitates activity and inactivity in some animals is the light/dark cycle. Richter studied the running activity of various species. The difference in running activity of rats with the lights on and off is shown in figure 2.4. A circadian clock is important for the onset of this behavior (Richter 1959b).

Circadian clocks orient and synchronize an animal's adaptive behavioral and physiological responses to periodic changes in the environment. The clock is a fundamental timing device expressed and present in a wide variety of species (Wehr et al. 1993). Richter studied the behavioral whole-organismic expression of circadian rhythmicity, believing in the independence of the clock from external and internal interference. His metaphor for the circadian clock was a wristwatch keeping time. Richter—mistakenly, it would turn out—believed that the circadian pacemaker was "free of all feedback" (Richter 1965; Rusak and Zucker 1979).

Richter provided an inquiry into the phenomenon, not a settled record of the facts. He noted that variation in hormonal levels affected both the estrous

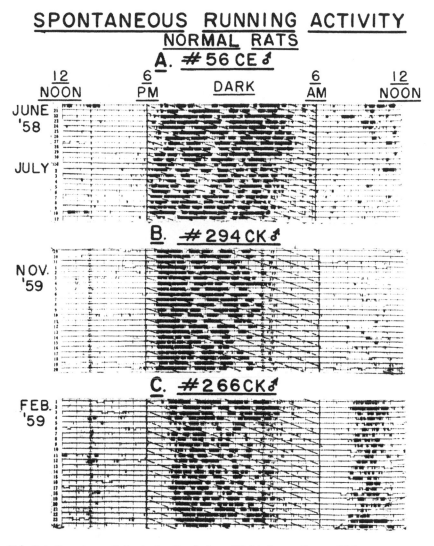

FIG. 2.4. Running activity during the dark and light phases. *Source:* Richter 1965

cycle and running activity in rats but mistakenly assumed that the clock could not be changed by this variation. Hormones can indeed affect the hard-wired expression of the circadian clock and alter the pattern itself; the hands of the clock can be changed somewhat by various hormones, such as estrogen (Morin, Fitzgerald, and Zucker 1977), or by activity or novelty alone (Mrosovsky and Janik 1993). Richter and his colleagues ablated many regions of the nervous system and determined the effects of these ablations on circadian rhythmicity. He approached his subjects from the purview of long-term studies, in some instances studying a subject and behavior over years.

Richter discovered that an ablation "somewhere in the hypothalamus" disrupted circadian rhythmicity. He reported that producing lesions on the hypothalamus resulted in disruption of circadian rhythms. Richter did not often present histology for his brain lesion inferences, but he did show one case in which a tumor disrupted circadian rhythmicity (Richter 1965).

Later it would become known that Richter had indeed been close to localizing the region of the brain essential for circadian rhythmicity when he noted that damage to the hypothalamus disrupted circadian rhythmicity (Richter 1965). In the early 1970s, two groups of investigators concurrently uncovered the essential role of the suprachiasmatic region (SCN) of the hypothalamus, which receives retinal information directly (Moore and Eichler 1972; Stephan and Zucker 1972). Richter himself reported that damage by a knife-cut in this region disrupted the regulation of behavior by the twenty-four-hour clock (Richter 1978a).

Richter was prescient, as were several of his colleagues (Aschoff, Gerecke, and Wever 1967; Aschoff 1981), to believe that the circadian clock was ancient and present in single cells. In fact, we know that many end-organ systems in the body have twenty-four-hour rhythms; for example, the activity of liver enzymes varies with the time of day. Richter was also prescient to suggest the independence of these clocks within several end-organ systems, both inside and outside the central nervous system, although damage to the SCN compromises some of the clocks' rhythmic patterns.

Richter suggested two types of sleep regulatory mechanisms, one linked to homeostatic requirements for sleep and the other to circadian rhythmic activity. He suggested that sleep activity was tied to the reticular formation and perhaps beholden to homeostatic needs (Richter 1967c).

How Many Clocks? Richter surmised that there were multiple clocks. A study of individual animals showed some variation in the clocks under normal conditions; these were further exaggerated under pathological conditions. He noted clocks in the Norway rat with cycles of 1–2 hours, 24 hours, 4–5 days, 12–14 days, 14–22 days, 30 days, 40–60 days, 76–124 days, and 160–180 days, and in other species, some with exceptional duration, like one in the chipmunk with a cycle of 6.5 years (Richter 1965). In fact, Richter's emphasis on individual differences, and perhaps his nonuse of statistical analysis, allowed him to pay more attention to this variation in clocks than many others in the field later would.

Richter noted variations in the adrenal glands of wild rats captured in different seasons. The adrenal glands of rats captured in the summer were smaller than those of rats captured during the early winter. The difference was more striking in males than in females. He claimed that male adrenal glands were 50 percent heavier in rats captured in the early winter than in rats captured in the summer (Rogers and Richter 1948).

Many studies have demonstrated seasonal clocks linked to hibernation and sexual activity. Variations in testosterone and luteinizing hormone concentration are linked to the seasons of spring and summer and to sexual reproduction activities (Nelson 1995). Seasonal physiological and behavioral changes in animals are commonplace and underlie many adaptations.

The Discovery of Fire. Richter had tagged the importance of the twenty-four-hour clock in a variety of species, noting species variation (whether the animals were nocturnal, etc.). The clocks were expressed by neonates and functioned to organize both behavior and physiology (Richter 1977a).

Richter held the view that human beings were less under the influence of circadian rhythmicity than other mammals because of inventions such as the use of fire. In some respects, this point of view reflected a variant of his view of domestication—the effects of cultural evolution on our internal organs.

Experiments in humans by Aschoff, Gerecke, and Wever found that men who remained in soundproof chambers and in constant light still displayed circadian rhythmicity (Aschoff, Gerecke, and Wever 1967). Despite these findings, Richter believed that under normal conditions, not extreme or pathological conditions, the twenty-four-hour clocks lay "submerged" in us, a piece of biological adaptation dormant in physiology and behavior. He certainly was wrong about the internal physiology. Many studies have shown that circadian rhythmicity underlies a variety of physiological functions in normal people. For example, variation in the light/dark cycle results in predictable changes in melatonin, prolactin, and other endocrine measures in many animals, including humans (Wehr et al. 1993). We did not lose this ability because of culture. Of course, cultural effects on biological adaptation were part of the underlying intellectual current for Richter and other investigators, principally Charles Darwin and William James.

With the control of light, our dependence on the internal twenty-four-hour clock became less important and less visible, except under conditions of pathology and emergency. Richter thought this was because of our cultural evolution. He commented that "probably the most important effect produced on early man was the great increases in waking hours" (Richter 1977a, p. 59). Further, he suggested that "these extra hours could be used for cultural and intellectual purposes" (Richter 1977a, p. 59). There was an interest in circadian clocks in Europe, but mostly those in plants and insects (Bunning 1963). Richter had the important insight that the biological clocks evident in plants and insects were also well represented in reptiles, birds, and mammals (Bunning 1963), and he added an interest in the regulation and expression of behavior and physiology. He inferred that great biological variants in adaptations to local niches figure in physiological and behavioral adaptations.

THE SHOCK-PHASE HYPOTHESIS

The shock-phase hypothesis is a biological hypothesis for the emergence of synchronicity as an adaptation. Richter offered this theory to account for the large expression of clocks or cycles. After an insult to the body, a new cyclic phenomenon emerges. Richter thought that bodily pathology reflected aberrations in the timing mechanism of circadian clocks and that, in humans, pathology allowed us to see clocks that were not normally revealed. A shock to the system invokes more synchronicity between organ cyclic phenomena, though it is important to distinguish shock effect from rhythmic patterns.

Do aberrations bring out more oscillatory responses? Yes, but we still don't know how many. Is the shock phase hypothesis warranted? According to Benjamin Rusak, a leading expert in the field, it is.

> Despite the lack of scientific interest in the shock-phase hypothesis for many years, an intriguing recent study lends some general support to the idea. A study of cultured fibroblasts demonstrated the emergence of several circadian cycles of gene expression in response to a single (hence, aperiodic) shock of high concentration serum delivered to the culture system. This observation suggests that even cells that appear to have no inherent rhythmicity may begin to express rhythms in response to a single external perturbation. It is possible that the external stimulus acted to synchronize rhythmic but asynchronous cells or to initiate rhythms in cells with an unexpressed potential for circadian rhythmicity. (Rusak 2000, p. 445)

TABLE 2.1. Conditions That May Bring Out Periodic Phenomena in Humans

Trauma	Debilitation
Vascular damage to brain	Thyroid deficiency
High fever	Cerebral arteriosclerosis
Brain tumor	Syphilis
Various illnesses	Parathyroid deficiency
Brain lesions	Severe stress or shock
Lethargic encephalitis	Food and other allergies

Source: Richter 1965

Richter documented a long list of clinical syndromes that were periodic and linked to bodily pathology. Some of the examples he noted were periodic bleeding, Hodgkin disease, Parkinsonian paresis, peptic ulcer, manic-depressive illness, sleep disturbances, and catatonic schizophrenia. Table 2.1 lists the conditions that may bring out periodic phenomena in humans (Richter 1965).

Richter's eye was on therapeutic goals (the clinical practical implications of basic biological research) as well as on normal functioning. He suggested, for example, links between parathyroid and calcium deficiency and depression and between thyroid deficiency and catatonic schizophrenia (Richter 1965). Richter noted parenthetically that "it must be made clear here that this was not a planned experiment" when he discussed some of his work on the effects of endocrine manipulations on rhythmic activity.

Richter compared the periodic catatonia observed by L. R. Gjessing with the effects of sulfametrazine administration on normal rats (Richter 1959b). The laboratory analogue suggested that thyroid hormone is a factor in the catatonic feature of schizophrenia and, Richter thought, that restoring thyroid balance brings a semblance of stability to the body and is fundamental in the organization of activity. Under different experimental conditions, Richter demonstrated how changes in thyroid function resulted in the expression of different cyclic patterns. Subsequent researchers have linked thyroid activation and the regulation of behavioral systems (McEachron and Schull 1993; Bauer, Heinz, and Whybrow 2002).

Richter had a long correspondence with L. R. Gjessing, whose lectures (Chesney Archives), revealed the influence of Richter's thinking. The periodic nature of illness—the fact that at different times of the day or week or month different physical symptoms become manifest and then recede into the background—was a clinical insight that permeated Richter's thinking about biological clocks (see Richter 1965 for more details about his work on clocks).

CONCLUSION

Richter's discovery that clocks are at the heart of the origins of animal activity and inactivity are quite profound. Richter the naturalist held fast to the real world. Richter the engineer tinkered with how to understand the machinations of the design of an internal system that codes and adapts to the environment.

But Richter the psychobiologist noted that "we have found great individual differences in the levels of activity" of the rat, and he suggested that the same holds for humans. He wrote that the endocrine glands were vital for maintaining "total energy expenditure" (Richter 1932, p. 353). Levels of human activity, he suggested, reflected the expression of a variety of endocrine output from the thyroid, adrenal glands, and gonads.

Cyclic internal machinations and the external environment are coordinated into an expression of adaptation. But because the internal milieu is separate from the external environment, active self-regulation lies at the center of our evolutionary landscape. Richter's ingenuity was to show the fundamental link between cyclic rhythms and their self-generation, the connection of the rhythms to the larger environment, and the origins of self-regulation.

Richter was always interested in biological clocks and thought that his psychobiological laboratory revealed something about the diversity of the clocks, including annual cyclicity or seasonal rhythms (e.g., Prendergast, Nelson, and Zucker 2002). But we did not lose our capacity for biological rhythmicity because we learned how to use fire and invented the light bulb. Our SCN did not atrophy; our pineal gland still secretes melatonin. The sense that our biological proclivities were undermined by our cultural advances, or at least that they could be, and that biological clocks were another instance of loss of biological function with advances in culture, was a misguided belief regarding both culture and biology.

Richter was supported in this research by several individuals, two of whom were particularly important. One, of course, was Meyer, and the other was Walter Cannon. Richter's research on clocks was supported in part by the National Research Council. Cannon was very much involved in monitoring Richter's work, including his observations on humans; in one letter to Cannon (Cannon Archives, Harvard University Press, March 1, 1943), Richter noted sadly that "in our work on the cyclic variation in psychiatric patients we had many disappointments, for during the past two years, possibly due to a very rapid turnover of patients, or just poor luck we have found very few who showed good behavior cycles."

In the same year, in Richter's annual report to the National Research Council (July 1942 to February 1943), he noted a fourteen-year-old patient who "showed very regular 40-day cycles in mood and behavior over a 6-month period." He also noted that there was no indication of any abnormality in the endocrine glands, nor any imbalance of mineral content, except somewhat for phosphorus. Richter, it seems, always had his eye on the patients in the clinic.

Richter made important and lasting contributions to the field of chronobiology, the study of the biological clocks that underlie physiology and behavior, though he may be less known than individuals who defined themselves solely in the context of this field (see Aschoff 1981). Because much of Richter's experimental focus was on blind animals, however, he overlooked the important role of the entrainment of clocks by events in the external world, adaptations, or synchronization to the external world.

How many clocks are there? As I have noted, Richter identified quite a number of them. Of course, the number depends on the animal species in question. The most plausible are the twenty-four-hour and the seasonal clocks, but other clocklike rhythmic patterns do exist and reflect the evolution of an organism and the terrain to which it has adapted.

Richter highlighted three features of clocks: those responsive to homeostatic changes, centrally generated pacemakers, and peripheral clocks. He thought homeostatic clocks were the least accurate, because they were subject to the effects of the environment. Central clocks clicked with precision, keeping perfect time. Peripheral clocks are associated with, for example, periodic swelling of a knee or lymphocyte production from the lymph gland. We now know, as Richter suggested, that both central and peripheral clocks are essential to bodily viability (Rosenwasser and Adler 1986; Rusak 2000).

Richter's love of clocks was lifelong and clinically oriented. The clinical manifestations of joint ailments, immune disorders, gastrointestinal distress, salivary secretions, and skin- and brain-related syndromes were all internally generated, he emphasized. Richter, still at it years later, published a paper in 1971 entitled "Inborn Nature of the Rat's 24-hour Clock," in which he demonstrated that the lack of visual sensibility does not deprive the rat of the inherent circadian rhythmicity (Richter 1971). The clocks are innate.

But Richter also emphasized variation and associated clinical syndromes with individual differences. His laboratory was an extension of the clinical ward. The goal of the laboratory was to simulate clinical syndromes in order to study them in detail. He sought to elucidate what turned activity on and off and then to discern its aberrations during pathological conditions—what Richter called "a biological approach to manic-depressive insanity" and other clinical syndromes (Richter 1930a). Richter noted changes in activity and inactivity that resulted from changes in glandular and neural function, work that had practical implications for the study of the role of clocks in depression and psychosis.

Richter's research into biological clocks was quite important; he was nominated for a Nobel Prize in 1981 for his work on "the biological clock as a timer in biology and behavior." Although he did not receive the prize, he achieved wide recognition for this work, which was only a part of his vast experimental contribution.

In the 1960s, research on the inherent nature of clocks in the regulation of behavior and physiology would explode (e.g., Aschoff and Wever 1965; Aschoff, Gerecke, and Wever 1967; Pittendrigh 1974; Aschoff 1981). Richter worked in isolation from what would eventually expand into a community of inquirers devoted to understanding the role of clocks. Perhaps he would have integrated what would become an important part of the idea of circadian clocks, entrainment to external events, if he had been less isolated from others in the field.

According to Irving Zucker, a noted investigator of biological clocks, "Richter may have been without peers in uncovering various rhythms in several species but the idiographic nature of some of his work, absence of tightly controlled, statistically evaluated experiments, diminished their impact, particularly post-1972, when many people joined an enterprise that Richter almost single-handedly kept alive for several decades. I was certainly stimulated and encouraged by his work" (I. Zucker, pers. comm., 2002).

Richter's obituary, which appeared in the *New York Times* on December 22, 1988, began: "Curt Richter, credited with the discovery of biological clocks, is dead at 94." He began his career with the clocks and thought about them until his death, and was heralded along the way for giving substance to the idea of the biological clock. Indeed, there is no doubt that he did just that. Was he right about everything? No. Was he correct about many features of the big picture? Absolutely!

CHAPTER 3

Ingestive Behaviors
and the Internal Milieu

Self-regulation of the internal milieu was a fundamental scientific subject for Curt Richter. He was not alone in this, but he was a major force in providing interesting and informative contexts in which to consider the biological adaptation required for bodily health. The internal milieu and its maintenance, or the concept of homeostasis (Cannon 1932/1966), was a fundamental category in his scientific lexicon.

Richter's work on the subject was a direct outgrowth of that of Bernard and Cannon. As Richter understood the work: "Both Bernard and Cannon concerned themselves almost entirely with the physiological and chemical regulators of the internal environment. The results of our own experiments have shown that behavior or total organism regulators also contribute to the maintenance of a constant internal environment" (Richter 1942–43, p. 64). Of course, the orientation toward the "total organism" is reminiscent of Adolf Meyer. These are the ideas Richter assumed, the culture of ideas he inherited and combined with a general sense of adaptation.

Another key concept for Richter was the ancient idea of self-preservation. Several hundred years before Darwin, Spinoza (1668/1955), in his great treatise *On the Improvement of the Understanding,* would make self-preservation fundamental to living entities (in long-lived organisms). Darwin (1859/1965) situated the concepts of self-preservation, self-regulation, and self-defense of internal viability within overall biology. Adaptation, speciation, diversity, and sexual dimorphism were all part of both behavior and physiology (Gould 2002).

REGULATION OF THE INTERNAL MILIEU
AND PHYSIOLOGICAL HOMEOSTASIS

Claude Bernard brought an experimental focus to the study of the internal milieu (Olmsted and Olmsted 1952; Holmes 1974). His logic of discovery centered on the functioning of biological tissue during normal conditions and under pathological duress. The body was indeed a "wonderful machine" for Bernard, and he focused his investigations on understanding bodily mechanisms.

Richter was clearly influenced by Bernard. Bernard's mentor, François Magendie, was the founder of experimental physiology and one of the first to use rodents in experimental physiology (Olmsted 1944; Holmes 1974; Wirth 1989). Among other things, Magendie was interested in pancreatic function and bodily responses to toxins. The logic of the experimental method in physiological studies was perhaps clarified by the work of William Harvey and was later expanded on by Magendie, Bernard, and many other investigators (Olmsted and Olmsted 1952; Holmes 1974).

Bernard's work on pancreatic function set the stage for investigations into the "chemistry of digestion" (Bernard 1856/1985, p. 1), which would be integral to understanding the maintenance of the internal milieu. These studies were performed in long-term experimental preparations (e.g., Pavlov 1897/1902; G. P. Smith 2000).[1] The idea of bodily regulation of the internal milieu did not originate with Richter; it was very much in the zeitgeist when he began to study it. Nor did it originate with Cannon, with whom we normally associate the phrase "wisdom of the body," but with a British physiologist, Ernest Starling (1923), in a lecture delivered to the Royal College of Physicians in London.[2]

CANNON AND BODILY REGULATION

Embodied in the concept of the "wisdom of the body" that Cannon inherited from Starling are the ways in which the body adapts to external circumstance and internal needs by generating physiological and behavioral responses. Cannon's experiments were mostly physiological, but he alluded to behavioral regulation, including the ingestion of sodium and calcium in the context of increased bodily needs. Behavioral regulation would figure in Richter's monumental contribution, behavioral homeostasis.

Cannon, in an early book entitled *Bodily Changes in Pain, Hunger, Fear and Rage,* outlined in some detail the physiology of adaptation under various conditions, including emotional conditions, hunger, and thirst. He criticized James for overassociating emotions with movement and for classifying the emotions as a function of, for example, running away from a bear. We can be afraid and not move. We can move or not—but fear is still there (Cannon 1915/1929).

The regulation of the adrenal gland and the enhanced use of glucose during duress figured prominently in Cannon's text. Cannon outlined a peripheralist perspective on thirst and hunger; he saw dry mouth and stomach contractions as the primary antecedents of thirst and hunger, respectively. For thirst, "the first state . . . there is a feeling of dryness in the mouth and throat, accompanied by a craving for liquid" (Cannon 1915/1929, p. 304).

Cannon (1932/1966), in his book *The Wisdom of the Body,* brought together many of his investigations, including research on body fluid homeostasis; thirst and hunger; and homeostatic regulation of salt, sugar, protein, fat, calcium, oxygen, blood, and temperature (Cannon 1932/1966). Each would figure in Richter's inquiry. Perhaps the individual who most influenced Richter's research was Walter Cannon.

In Cannon's words: "The constant conditions which are manifested in the body might be termed equilibria. That word, however, has come to have a fairly exact meaning applied to relatively simple physio-chemical states, in closed systems, where known forces are balanced. The coordinated physiological processes which maintain most of the steady states in the organism are so complex and so peculiar to living beings—involving as they may, the brain and nerves, the heart, lungs, kidneys and spleen, all working cooperatively— that I have suggested a special designation for these states, homeostasis" (Cannon 1932/1966, p. 24). A little later, Cannon said, "It means a condition— a condition which may vary but which is relatively constant" (p. 24). In other words, homeostasis is the key to keeping the internal milieu viable, maintaining levels of glucose, and secreting adrenaline. Cannon's studies in physiology were quite broad and set the stage for Richter. Richter was much influenced by Cannon's perspective on hunger and fluid balance but noted that the brain generates the behavioral adaptations (Richter 1956d).

As noted in chapter 2, Richter found evidence linking patterns of activity and inactivity in rats to stomach contractions. And while he was not wrong to emphasize the stomach, the activation of the stomach is but one peripheral signal among others participating in the regulation of food ingestion (Friedman et al. 1985; G. P. Smith 1997).

Cannon also influenced Richter's work on the biological basis of food choice. After all, on several occasions Cannon noted that behavior serves physiology, that animals are likely to ingest calcium during pregnancy, when the need for calcium is great, and that bone and other tissue suffer the consequences of calcium deficiency. Cannon also suggested that animals might ingest sodium during periods of sodium deficiency (Cannon 1932/1966). Cannon laid the seeds for a view of behavioral regulation of the internal milieu; Richter's contribution was to expand considerably beyond Cannon's physiological perspective and show that behavior serves physiology in this regulation. No one had, or has, demonstrated this in the laboratory as elegantly as Richter. By 1941, Richter, in an essay entitled "Biology of Drives," would assert that "Bernard and Cannon dealt largely with the physiological regulators—responses of individual organs or systems—which serve to maintain a constant internal environment. Several years ago we found that the organism itself, the total organism, may also play an important part" (Richter 1941c, p. 105).

INSTINCT, BEHAVIOR, AND PSYCHOBIOLOGY

Instinct was a fundamental psychobiological category for Richter, and he saw behavior, and in particular the behavioral regulation of the internal milieu, as falling chiefly under this rubric. The concept was understood differently by different investigators.[3] There was no univocal notion of instinct, but it was (and still is) an important concept, one fundamental to Richter's scientific lexicon. Instinctive behaviors explained how animals select the nutrients and minerals needed to maintain physiological viability.

Instinct figured importantly for Darwin (1873). The issue that permeated biology and psychobiology in his day was the relationship between inherited and acquired traits. Darwin was prescient when he said, "I will not attempt any definition of instinct" (Darwin 1859/1965, p. 228). Always the consummate empiricist, Darwin gave examples of what he thought were migratory, sexual, and social instincts. He thought that domestication diminished the effectiveness of instinctive behaviors. For example, through domestication fowls became less "broody," spending less time sitting on their eggs.

Darwin noted that species-specific behavioral and physiological adaptations were richly expressed and perhaps tied to finding sources of energy and to primary motivational systems and their release in suitable environments; this was a precursor to later studies on animal behavior and ethology (Beer 1983; Craig 1918; Tinbergen 1951/1969).

Darwin, like many others, was unclear about "habits" and their link to instincts and about new instincts emerging from domestication. Throughout his writings, Darwin remained a gradualist with regard to evolutionary selection based on the emergence of instincts. He acknowledged that "instincts are not always perfect" (Darwin 1859/1965, p. 256). After all, he understood problem solving as not about perfection but about adaptation. In the *Descent of Man,* he went on to compare our evolution with that of other species and suggested that "the fewness and the comparative simplicity of the instincts in the higher animals are remarkable in contrast with those of the lower animals" (Darwin 1871/1874, p. 65).

The concept of instinct in Darwin's time, and for a hundred years afterward, was rich in multiple and confusing meanings (Beer 1983). Issues about what was heritable and the battle for Lamarckian transmission permeated the debates (Darwin 1859/1965; Morgan 1910; J. L. Gould 2002). Many ideas surround the concept of instinct, but one fundamental feature has always been the dichotomy between the inherited and the learned, or the distinction between innate and learned behaviors. Of course, it need not have been so controversial because learning is part of our innate endowment, as is adaptation to varied environments. The modern question is which behavioral systems are being recruited, and to what degree. For when intelligence is part of adaptation and of instinctive behaviors, distinctions fizzle away; the question is degree, not kind.

James, in an unusually harsh tone, wrote that "the older writing on instinct is an ineffectual waste of words" (James 1887, p. 356). Some consensus centered on the idea that instincts were reflexive responses to characteristic stimuli (cf. James 1887; Watson 1912). James, though somewhat inconsistently, thought that "instinct is usually defined as the faculty of acting in such a way as to produce certain ends without foresight" (James 1890/1952, p. 383; see also Epstein 1982). An instinct reflected sets of impulses and reflexes. One of James's examples of this was the reflexes involved in egg laying.

The sense of being hostage to instinct, blindly performing functions tied to natural selection, is a recurrent theme in the literature about instinct (cf. Epstein 1982; James 1887), as is "the close relation of instinct to reflex action" (James 1887, 1890/1952; Herrnstein 1972). The concept of a reflex became a pivotal part of characterizing instinctive responses (Herrnstein 1972). Reflexes were the way many mechanists understood how to generate a psychology based on science.

As Herrnstein made clear, at some points early in Watson's career his view on instinct was not dissimilar to James's view (Herrnstein 1972; Dewsbury 1992). Though Watson commented that "we have been brought up on James or possibly even on a worse diet" (Watson 1924, p. 110), early on, Watson provided examples of several contexts in which the concept of instinct had validity (Watson 1912; Yerkes 1903). But he also noted the variability of behavioral responses and the effects of altering early environments and minimizing instinctive responses. For example, Watson asserted that the normal fear responses of several species of birds could be suppressed by environmental events. Moreover, he challenged the notion that all behaviors, even those in which there is a biological basis, are adaptive (Watson 1912). Watson may have retained the idea that other animals had instincts, but he was interested only in humans. Therefore, Watson, under the ideological spell of behaviorism, rejected the concept of instinct; as he put it, "There are then for us no instincts. We no longer need the term in psychology" (Watson 1924, p. 94). One behaviorist practice, which would be Skinner's practice, was to apply Occam's razor to the science of behavior; no mental entities have real legitimacy. There was no "inheritance of traits," as Watson would put it; temperament, for example, could not be inherited.

But in a very real sense, instincts are to psychobiology what phrenology is to neurology, and this has resulted in a very long, complicated, and confusing literature. McDougall's (1910) work is but one example. The central questions of this period were: How many instincts can there be? What is the definition of an instinct? What are the constraints for using the concept of instinct?

The fight for legitimacy and coherence of the concept of instinct went back and forth in both North America and Europe. Throughout this fight, there were those who attempted to clarify the concept of instinct and those who primarily rejected it, the latter including Knight Dunlap, the nominal head of Richter's committee in psychology and a close colleague of Watson. Dunlap felt that the concept of instinct should be replaced with a discussion of "instinctive activities" (Dunlap 1919).

Karl Lashley, in his influential article "Experimental Analysis of Instinctive Behavior," noted that he was "well aware that instincts were banished from psychology some years ago, but that purge seems to have failed" (Lashley 1938/1960). The article defended a view of central states in which the brain underlies the periodic behavior that fascinated Richter. In that same paper, Lashley commented on the work of Richter and his colleagues, reminding the community that stomach contractions are not the primary source of motivation to ingest food. In other words, although the contractions may have been rhythmic and linked to hunger, the instinctive and motivational responses were not. Lashley noted that the problem of motivation was closely linked to that of instinctive behavior and sensory-motor control (Stellar 1954).

Richter assumed that the concept of instinct was fundamental to understanding the specific hungers. And he found a variety of ways in which instinctive behavioral responses serve physiological viability. In other words, Richter understood that behavioral regulation of nutritional choice, the so-called wisdom of the body, and the internal milieu were central to the study of instinctive or innate adaptive responses.

INNATE NUTRITIONAL CHOICE

The intellectual climate Richter inhabited held that nutritional choice and bodily regulation were an apparent piece of biological design. Studies showed that a variety of species could select proteins, carbohydrates, and perhaps even vitamins when they were needed. In 1915, for example, Evvard reported that when swine were offered a set of nine food choices, they displayed adequate growth rates. Osborne and Mendel offered rats diets with balanced or unbalanced amino acid content and reported that the rats selected the balanced diets (Osborne and Mendel 1918).

Anecdotal observations noted in print since the eighteenth century had reported that cattle tended to ingest bone. This was interpreted as possibly reflecting a phosphorus deficiency, representing a specific appetite (Green 1925; Denton 1982). In this biological context, animals approached and avoided objects of specific nutritional value, behaviors that reflected appetitive and consummatory responses (Craig 1918).

Clara Davis studied the choice of nutrients by humans at Children's Memorial Hospital in Chicago (Davis 1928, 1935, 1939). She offered infants from six to eleven months of age, who were recently weaned and had not been exposed to "ordinary foods of adult life" (Davis 1939), a large assortment of nutritional sources. The fresh foods were prepared daily and included sweet milk, peaches, lamb, kidney, wheat, potatoes, peas, beets, and cabbage. The thirty-four food sources were not offered at the same time, but different foods were offered in separate dishes three to four times a day. Davis found that the infants selected a diet that was adequate to maintain bodily viability. She reported that the infants gained body weight and looked healthy over the duration of the test.

One could not imagine doing these experiments today. (Imagine getting by an institutional review board with this research plan.) The rationale was to look at infants at the time they were weaned and determine the adequacy of their early choices. Davis found satisfactory nutrition in most of her subjects, although not all. When four of the infants became undernourished and five appeared to have rickets, these infants were removed from the study. Davis's studies endorsed the concept of the wisdom of the body. Davis suggested that "some innate, automatic mechanism" was operative (1939, p. 260), but because she varied the diet, she also cogently suggested that there was "trial and error sampling." A caveat, however, accompanies what she calls "trial and error methods," namely, the "fallibility of appetite" (1939, p. 261). She then suggests that "there is no instinct pointing blindly to the food." However, what cannot be determined from the Davis experiments are (1) how many combinations or choices would have given a positive result and what was the minimum of choices necessary to accomplish a positive result, and (2) what was the likelihood that offering a random, well-balanced selection of foods would result in a similar outcome.

Richter thought that ingestive behavior reflected innate structure. He stepped into a rich cultural intellectual milieu that was centered around the question of adaptive versus nonadaptive nutritional choice behaviors. An intellectual debate was taking place over issues concerning innate and learned influences on behavior, and Richter would weigh in very heavily on one side. His model of behavioral control was created from the standpoint of a biological engineer. He asked the question, "What structure of behavior ensures an adequate supply of nutrients and minerals for internal viability?" Innate structure figured prominently in this model.

Richter's approach was constant and predictable in retrospect. Remove an organ (often in a surgical tour de force), understand the physiological effects of that removal, and provide opportunities for animals to restore physiological viability through behavior. For example, there was a long and varied context for studying pancreatic function in the use and digestion of foods and fuel sources (e.g., Bernard 1856/1985; Pavlov 1897/1902). Richter and his colleagues added behavioral regulation as a fundamental part of the analysis of adaptation.

McCOLLUM AND THE CORE DIET

The diets for most of Richter's studies were derived from the work of E. V. McCollum, a noted biochemist and nutritionist at Hopkins. Richter looked to the work of his colleague for instruction in preparing diets. The McCollum diet included, among other foods, graham flour, skim milk powder, casein, butter, calcium carbonate, and salt.

BODY FLUID BALANCE: WATER AND SODIUM REGULATION

Richter thought that the excessive water intake resulting from diabetes insipidus was primarily due to polyuria (Richter 1935). The concept of body fluid regulation arose from the knowledge that water and sodium disturbances were often linked.

In experiments Richter and others observed that damage to the pituitary gland that interfered with vasopressin (ADH) secretion resulted in a compromised capacity to regulate water balance. The normal response, when dehydrated or depleted of extracellular fluid, is to conserve water through the kidney via the secretion of ADH from the pituitary. The rats in Richter's experiments ingested more water than usual. The behavior of water ingestion that normally occurs with dehydration was exaggerated in the animals in which ADH secretion was compromised. Richter concluded that behavior played a large role in maintaining internal viability. Rats drank water as a compensatory response when physiological water regulation became less competent.

Richter selected an important entry to the study of ingestive behavior, the behavioral regulation of sodium. It had been known that adrenalectomy resulted in the depletion of sodium and in potential death and that if sodium levels returned to normal, longevity increased. Cannon and others had suggested, based on anecdotal observations, that "animals travel long distances to salt licks to satisfy their hunger." Cannon added, "The nature of this hunger is quite unknown" (Cannon 1932/1966, p. 96).

Richter's insight was to add sources of sodium to the diets of adrenalectomized rats and study them using the "appetite method," as he liked to call it. When offered a range of choices, rats always ingested sodium of several concentrations in greater amounts than other solutes. Rats were often studied over a considerable period of time, and there was always normative baseline data (in this case, the ingestion of the various solutes by non-adrenalectomized rats) with which to compare the effects of the experimental manipulations (fig. 3.1). In many of the studies, Richter offered sodium solutions individually or with a range of other solutes and plain water.

Richter noted a range of ingestive patterns heavily biased toward sodium solutes when animals were hungry for sodium, as many other investigators

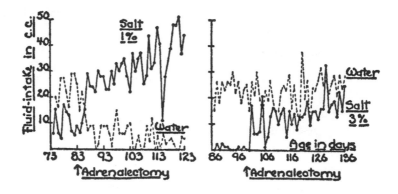

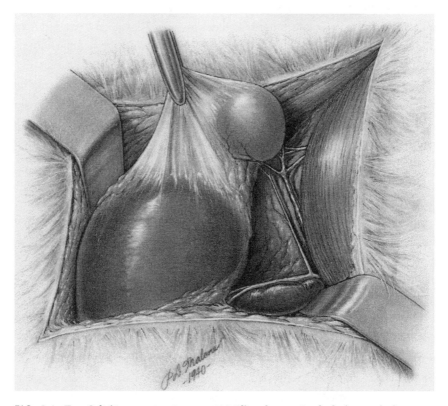

FIG. 3.1. *Top:* Salt (1 percent or 3 percent NaCl) and water intake before and after adrenalectomy. Note the increase in salt intake after adrenalectomy. *Bottom:* The adrenal gland being removed from a rat. *Source:* Richter 1936a, 1941h

have also noted (e.g., Wolf 1969; Schulkin 1991). He also noted that when the adrenal tissue was transplanted, sodium ingestion returned to normal in several of the animals studied because the rats were no longer excreting sodium in excessive amounts.

These experiments, and many others performed by Richter and his colleagues, demonstrated that "the fact that the adrenalectomized rats made advantageous selections from the various chemical solutions offered brings further evidence for the validity of Cannon's concept of the wisdom of the body" (Richter and Eckert 1938).

Richter observed that several of the animals immediately ingested the sodium when it was offered, and he suggested that adrenalectomy-induced sodium loss resulted in an innate specific appetite for sodium, something others would later demonstrate in great detail (e.g., Epstein and Stellar 1955; Wolf 1969; Denton 1982; Schulkin 1991).

Richter noted that salt and water ingestion had an inverse relationship with diabetes and, importantly, that when adrenal tissue was restored the adrenalectomized subjects decreased their intake of sodium, presumably because they could now retain it. When deoxycorticosterone was given to rats with intact adrenal glands, the ingestion of sodium increased over baseline conditions; this suggested that mineralocorticoid regulation was knotted to the behavioral in addition to the physiological regulation of sodium. It was known that water intake increased with injections of deoxycorticosterone, and this was construed as a link to a diabetes insipidus–like syndrome. Katherine Rice and Richter wanted to determine whether water intake decreased when subjects were also given a sodium solution. What were rats really interested in ingesting? Richter alternately varied the content of sodium in the diet and access to water and sodium solutions and found that polydipsia (excessive water drinking) was dependent on sodium and that the appetite for sodium was primary (Rice and Richter 1943).

Indeed, loss of sodium (and elevation of the hormones of sodium homeostasis) trigger an appetite for sodium the very first time sodium salts are encountered (Nachman 1962; Wolf 1969). This was a major tenet of Richter's and has been tested over the last sixty years in many contexts. There are disputes about the degree of specificity, but nearly every investigator agrees that the first time a sodium-hungry animal is exposed to a sodium salt it immediately ingests the salt (Wolf 1969). In such instances, sodium ingestion is relatively specific for sodium salts and occurs too quickly for the consequences of the ingestion (absorption from the gut) to factor in the rats' immediate ingestion.

Richter described the choices offered in his typical experiments with rats and, of course, the cages in which the diets were provided. In one experiment, the rats were given seventeen choices. They preferred the sodium salt to a considerable degree. They ingested other salts, but not nearly as much as the sodium salts. When salts were offered alone, the ingestion of different concentrations of salt varied depending on the circumstance.

When rendered hungry for sodium by adrenalectomy, the rats ingested more sodium than usual; when the hormone deoxycorticosterone was implanted to the chamber of the eye, the rats' sodium intake normalized because replacing this sodium-retaining hormone halted sodium excretion. Deoxycorticosterone has both mineralocorticoid and glucocorticoid components. Rice and Richter (1943) showed that the mineralocorticoid at higher doses raised the ingestion of sodium salts preferentially over other salt solutions. Years later, others would demonstrate that aldosterone (e.g., Wolf 1964), the naturally occurring mineralocorticoid, had many of the same effects on behavior and physiology that Richter had noted with deoxycorticosterone and that the appetite for sodium is innate (cf. Weisinger and Woods 1971; Schulkin 1978).

Richter suggested that changes in the oral cavity, particularly in the gustatory system, contribute to the search for and ingestion of sodium salts when needed. In other words, the gustatory system plays a major role in the recognition of salt and the release of the consummatory response; an innate recognition or instinctual response underlies this. Richter determined, in both rats and humans, the gustatory thresholds for detecting various salts.

In one experiment, Richter offered adrenalectomized rats different concentrations of sodium salts to determine at what concentration they would prefer the sodium salt over water. Ingestion from the sodium bottle and the water bottle was determined to be about the same before the onset of the experimental manipulation (adrenalectomy). Thereafter, Richter observed the amount of sodium ingested relative to the amount of water ingested from the water and sodium bottles (offered in ascending concentrations). He suggested 0.055 percent NaCl as the concentration at which sodium-hungry rats begin to ingest more sodium salt than water (Richter 1936a, 1939a).

Richter and Alice MacLean would also do experiments in humans on gustatory responses to sodium. They placed different concentrations of NaCl in a dropper, the "drop method" or "swallow method," for normal, non-sodium-hungry people to taste. They found that the concentration at which subjects noticed the salt taste was close to that at which the sodium-hungry rats demonstrated their sodium-seeking behavior (Richter and MacLean 1939).

Richter suggested that changes in the oral cavity played an important role in sodium regulation. Other investigators would later do more sophisticated taste psychophysics on gustatory detection thresholds in both rats and humans (e.g., Bartoshuk 1974; Spector 2000), but this basic important role of the gustatory system in the regulation of sodium ingestion was accepted. Richter also experimented with cutting all three gustatory nerves in rats and observing compromised salt ingestion (Richter 1942–43, 1956d). Later investigators would show that the chorda tympani nerve is the cranial nerve most linked to the detection of the salt taste (e.g., Pfaffmann 1967; Contreras 1977).

In an article published in 1956, and in a section titled "Salt Appetite as a Regulator of Homeostasis," Richter began, "Bernard and Cannon have shown that mammals are endowed with a number of physiological mechanisms for the maintenance of the constancy of the internal environment. This includes among other things, keeping the composition of the body fluids within exceedingly narrow limits" (Richter 1956d, p. 616). The first sentence in the next paragraph asserted that that "behavioral mechanisms also help to maintain homeostasis is clearly demonstrated by our own experiments" (p. 618). To my mind, this essay is Richter's most elegant statement of his research. In it, Richter remained close to the source of his ideas. He never strayed far, and why should he? The ideas had scientific worth and productivity written into their history.

Always with an eye for the clinical, and to legitimate total self-regulatory behavior, Lawson Wilkins and Richter noted that a three-and-a-half-year-old child with adrenal pathology ingested large amounts of table salts (Wilkins and Richter 1940). This behavior was reported by the parents of the child, who stated that "there was no other one food that he seemed to crave like salt except water." The child showed intense interest in and ingestion of salt. By contrast, he avoided sweet substances. The parents said, tragically, that "even in his sickly condition" the child was very bright and paid attention in detail to the foods offered him at home. When placed on a normal diet in a hospital setting, the child died.

Influenced by the work of Davis, Richter understood this individual case to be an analogue of the adrenalectomized rat's craving for sodium. In other words, Wilkins and Richter interpreted this as another instance of behavior serving physiology in the maintenance of body sodium balance.

CALCIUM HOMEOSTASIS

When Richter turned to the study of calcium homeostasis, he approached the problem in the same manner as he had the study of sodium. First he demonstrated a calcium appetite, and then he suggested that ingestion behavior was organized by an innate capacity to detect calcium salts and triggered by decreased levels of calcium.

Again, the experimental method was the removal of specific tissue that would threaten calcium metabolism and absorption. In this case, Richter removed rats' parathyroid glands. The loss of calcium was life threatening. McCollum, his colleague at Hopkins, had done work on calcium deprivation and the link to rickets and tetany (e.g., McCollum et al. 1922; McCollum 1964). And importantly, Cannon had indicated that, although calcium is needed at all times, there are certain times for a female "when the demand for calcium is especially great. During pregnancy she must provide calcium for the developing fetus and throughout the months of nursing she must provide an even greater amount in the milk" (Cannon 1932/1966, p. 140).

Once again, as he nearly always did, Richter adapted the McCollum low-calcium diet to his own interests. He then offered the parathyroidectomized rats different calcium solutions mixed in water, along with a separate bottle of plain water. In further experiments, he offered them conjointly a range of calcium and other mineral solutions to determine which the rats would ingest. Although he did find that calcium was generally the more consumed mineral product, other solutions were ingested on occasion, including strontium and magnesium, whereas phosphate solutions tended to be avoided (Richter and Eckert 1937b; Richter and Helfrick 1943).

Richter and his colleagues also noted that high calcium content added back to the diet reduced the intake of calcium solutions by the parathyroidectomized rats (Richter and Birmingham 1941) or monkeys (Richter, Honeyman, and Hunter 1940). The method of removing a gland and then reinstating the tissue elsewhere was part of Richter's elegant laboratory expertise and artistry, and he demonstrated that only a small part of the tissue was needed to reinstate function. He reattached parts of the parathyroid to the eye to cause the parathyroid hormone to act as a calcium-retaining hormone. When this was done, the behavior of calcium ingestion was no longer as prevalent (fig. 3.2). When parathyroidectomized rats were injected with parathyroid extracts,

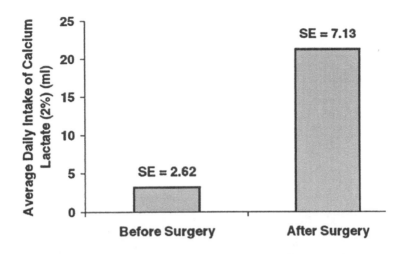

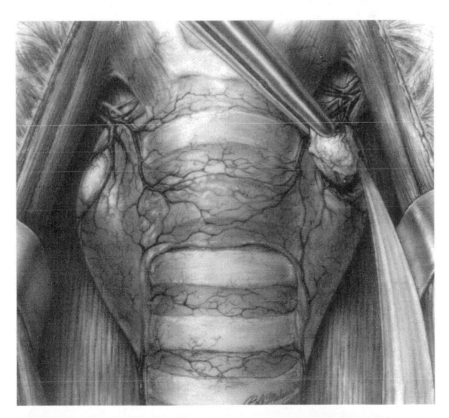

FIG. 3.2. *Top:* Calcium intake before and after parathyroidectomy. Note the change in calcium intake after surgery. *Bottom:* The parathyroid gland being removed from a rat. *Source:* Richter and Birmingham 1941

their calcium intake was also reduced (see also Richter and Birmingham 1941). Since Richter's time, the effects of the parathyroidectomy on calcium ingestion have been confirmed by a number of investigators (e.g., Leshem, Delcancho, and Schulkin 1999; Tordoff 2001).

The degree of specificity in calcium ingestion is still debatable (Leshem, Delcancho, and Schulkin 1999; Tordoff 2001). What is not debatable is that behavior toward calcium salts is altered by the level of calcium in the body, whether that level is reached by ingestion, intubation, or other means. And there is evidence that the appetite for calcium is innate (Leshem, Delcancho, and Schulkin 1999; Tordoff 2001).

PANCREATIC DAMAGE AND EXPERIMENTAL DIABETES

Richter noted that activity patterns were reduced in pancreas-damaged rats and inferred that this might be due to their insufficient capacity to use carbohydrates (Richter and Schmidt 1939, 1941). In several experiments, he and his colleagues ablated rats' pancreases and then determined the long- and short-term choice patterns of the rats. The rats' water intake was elevated by a number of dietary conditions. Richter made two sets of essential observations. One was that the rats avoided carbohydrates. Richter assumed that animals avoided what they could not use and what was health threatening. The elevated level of glucose in their plasma was part of the reason the rats drank more water and, Richter noted, was a result of their diet. The second important phenomenon Richter observed was enhanced oil ingestion by the rats. In further tests with varied diets, Richter and his colleagues expanded their findings of carbohydrate aversion and enhanced oil appetite in the pancreas-ablated rat (Richter, Schmidt, and Malone 1945) (fig. 3.3).

Richter and Schmidt also observed that insulin administration ameliorated the diabetic effects of pancreatic ablation, causing rats to reduce their intake of olive oil and begin ingesting sucrose in greater amounts. Subsequent studies would corroborate and extend Richter's findings by demonstrating that dietary manipulations affect oil and carbohydrate acceptability (Friedman et al. 1985).

Richter, Schmidt, and Malone (1945) described the case of Walter Fleischmann, an investigator and physician from Vienna who worked at the Harriet Lane Home for Invalid Children at Johns Hopkins Hospital. Fleischmann reported that, instead of using insulin, he kept his mild diabetes under control by ingesting lard. Fleischmann, interestingly, was also part of the original group that observed the young boy who ingested salt to compensate for adre-

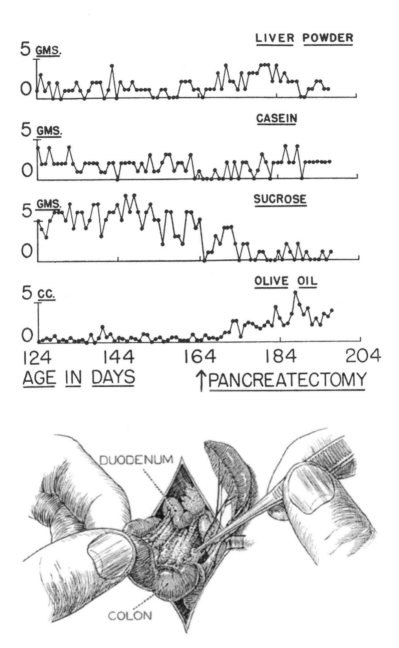

FIG. 3.3. *Top:* Ingestion patterns before and after pancreatectomy. Note the increase in oil intake following surgery. *Bottom:* The pancreas being removed from a rat. *Source:* Richter and Schmidt 1941; Richter, Schmidt, and Malone 1945

nal insufficiency. It is quintessential Richter to make the connection between the adrenal-damaged child ingesting table salt and the use of lard or fat by a mild diabetic.

THIAMINE AND VITAMIN B1 DEFICIENCY

Richter and other investigators (Harris et al. 1933) noted that vitamin B deficiency resulted in behaviors that could ameliorate the need for the vitamin. In Richter's experiment, he offered rats a cafeteria selection of foods and solutions and found that they seized on the source of the vitamin they needed. One method of eliciting a vitamin B deficiency was to eliminate yeast from the diet. The vitamin B–deficient animals decreased their intake of both carbohydrate and protein and increased their fat intake, which was adaptive because fats spare thiamine (Rozin 1976b). In subsequent analyses (Richter, Holt, and Barelare 1937a; Richter and Hawkes 1941), the lack of thiamine was found to be critical for carbohydrate and protein aversion and fat appetite (see also Scott and Verney 1949).

In further experiments, Richter noted that vitamin B–deficient rats ingested all of the solutions available containing B vitamins such as thiamine and riboflavin. Richter noted on several occasions that, although protein was actively ingested by normal rats on a self-selection regimen, vitamin B–deficient rats tended to avoid the protein when the same regimen was offered.

Richter wrote of an essential moment in an experiment with vitamin B: "One vitamin deficient rat drank 11cc or 5,500 international units, in less than half an hour; another rat drank 29cc, or 14,500 international units, in 24 hours" (Rozin 1967). Richter noted that the vitamin B–deficient animal was quite interested in the solutions. "This is shown by the fact that the rats found the bottles at once, even when as many as 12 different other containers filled with different food or solutions were present in the cage at the same time. It was difficult to stop the animals from drinking the substance once they had tasted it" (Richter, Holt, and Barelare 1937a; Rozin 1967, p. 413). Again, Richter, Holt, and Barelare observed that "the animals showed an immediate liking for the vitamin" and, in contrast to Harris and his group (Harris et al. 1933), suggested that the behavior "may not depend entirely on the experiences of a beneficial effect resulting from the ingestion of the vitamin" (Richter, Holt, and Barelare 1937a, p. 355).

Richter and Barelare reported that vitamin B–deficient rats did not ingest protein and sucrose but did ingest oil when it was offered in a self-selection context. The rats also ingested the thiamin and riboflavin, in addition to other vitamin B components (Richter and Barelare 1939a). Years later, in a letter to Paul Rozin, Richter noted subsequent variability and inconsistency in the vitamin B1–deficient rats' ingestive behavior. In Richter's words, "Let me tell you at once that I have never been able to repeat Barelare and my observations on well over 200 rats. For our original experiments we used natural B1, for all the other experiments we used synthetic preparations. This may in some way account for the discrepancy."

Richter continued, "In a few experiments I believe that we were able to experimentally produce changes in B1 appetite, but in most instances the results showed little consistency." He then noted parenthetically that "some of our best results were obtained—if my memory does not deceive me—from our so called single food choice experiments in which we offered the rats one food source" (personal files of Paul Rozin, University of Pennsylvania, July 11, 1963).

Clear from this line of research, and now well demonstrated, was the adaptive behavior that Richter and others (Barnett 1956; Rozin 1967) observed of ingesting feces as a means of conserving valuable vitamins and other sources of nutrients and minerals. When vitamin B–deficient rats were offered a bowl of feces in addition to other vitamin and nutritional sources, they ingested the feces at a greater rate than did rats that were not B-deficient.

Richter was less certain about the behavioral mechanisms of vitamin B–specific hunger (Harris et al. 1933; Scott 1946; Scott and Verney 1949), and he acknowledged that some form of trial-and-error learning may have been at work (Rozin 1967, 1976b). Investigators building on Richter's insights determined specific behavioral adaptations, such as sampling one food at a time, and then determined the consequences of vitamin B ingestion in the thiamine-deficient rats. Another behavioral mechanism at work was tagging novelty, keeping track of what was new (Rozin 1967, 1976b). The conclusion: there is no innate appetite for thiamine. When thiamine-deficient rats are offered choices of foods they switch to any novel diet rather than continuing to eat the diet that is rendering them ill. The investigators' finding that the rats had learned an aversion to the thiamine-deficient diet would serve as a model for studying other specific hungers (Rozin 1967, 1976b).

SELF-SELECTION OF NUTRIENTS UNDER VARIOUS EXPERIMENTAL CONDITIONS

Richter determined the survival rate of rats that consumed various metabolic fuels. To establish the optimal nutrient sources, he would offer rats a single item from his array of fats, carbohydrates, and proteins and then determine how long the rats survived on that single item. He then used the superior nutrient sources for his self-selection experiments (Richter, Holt, and Barelare 1937a). His paradigm guaranteed experimental success. This sounds like experimental good sense, except if it turns out the results are artifactual to the design rather than indicative of a real phenomenon (see Rozin and Schulkin 1990; Galef 1991). When Richter embarked on these studies, there existed a history of related experimentation using various animals to describe how appropriate nutritional choices are made (e.g., Evvard 1915).

As Richter understood it, he had already demonstrated successful behavioral adaptation to sodium and calcium deficiency. Now he would demonstrate that rats would select appropriate nutritional sources under general conditions. Rats were adapted to the McCollum diet, their ingestive patterns were determined, and then the diet was switched to a selection of the nutrient sources Richter had found optimal.

Richter used the self-selection apparatus in several metabolic and nutritional contexts (e.g., Richter 1943, 1956d). After determining the survival rate from the ingestion of various metabolic fuels and choosing the fuels with the maximal combination of minerals and vitamins, Richter offered eleven pure substances (casein, sucrose, olive oil, sodium chloride, dibasic sodium phosphate, calcium lactate potassium chloride, dried baker's yeast, cod liver oil, wheat germ oil, and water) in separate containers. Richter found that rats displayed the same normal growth on the self-selection diet that they did on the McCollum standardized diet. He also noted that the self-selection diet had a slightly lower total nutritional content than the McCollum diet, but the data suggested competence and achievement in nutritional intake regardless. Moreover, he demonstrated that one essential behavior was intact: the rats reproduced normally. Richter was not alone in his self-selection observations; disagreement surrounded the findings at that time, but only in terms of the extent to which the behavior was innate or learned.

Richter believed his experiments demonstrated innate organization in response to bodily needs (Richter 1943, 1956d). He asserted that rats have special appetites for a wide range of substances, including sodium, carbohydrates, protein, calcium, and phosphorus, in addition to various vitamins. Some of these assumptions would be challenged (e.g., Rozin, 1976b). How many innate appetites were there? Moreover, in the cafeteria context, did the rats really go into deficiency? If a need state could be considered on a moment-to-moment basis, could not Richter argue that they were never truly deficient because they were able to select the appropriate nutrients before a deficiency status was reached? Or did they manage to select the appropriate foods because only the optimal nutritional choices were offered? Did this simplify the context enough that, as in the Davis experiments with neonates (1928, 1935, 1939), the experiment was destined for success?

In some similar studies normal growth and adequate self-selection were achieved; in other studies they were not (e.g., Lat 1967). One view expressed by an insightful critic of the self-selection experiments was that it worked best when the diets were maximally nutritious (Galef 1991; see also Davis 1939). Moreover, the environmental context mattered; the way the foods were offered and their nutritional value were important experimental manipulations (Galef 1991). Richter did not vary in great detail the environmental context for self-selection.

Richter next turned his attention to pregnancy and lactation. Figure 3.4 reveals that ingestion of some substances, including sodium chloride and calcium lactate, increased during pregnancy or lactation. Richter noted that water intake was particularly elevated during lactation.

Carbohydrate and sucrose intake did not change during rats' reproductive periods. Moreover, Richter noted that caloric intake started out at 45.3 kcal before mating, rose to 59.8 kcal toward the end of pregnancy, peaked at 160.0 kcal during lactation, and then returned to 52.3 kcal after weaning. This general trend in caloric intake has been documented by others and demonstrated in humans; we also know that this trend varies from species to species and between women in Western and non-Western countries (Prentice 1994).

Richter was confident about the sodium, calcium, and phosphate demands of pregnancy, and the elevated intake of a variety of substances has now been well documented (Denton 1982). It is still not clear, however, to what extent the elevated intake of substances reflects the activation of specific innate regulatory needs rather than general ingestive patterns, such as a tendency to increase ingestion of a variety of (but not all) substances. The magnitude of the effects and the extent to which they have been confirmed have varied in the literature (e.g., Denton 1982; Woodside and Millelire 1987; Thiels, Verbalis, and Stricker 1990).

There is evidence that a number of hormones that are elevated during the reproductive periods, some of which Richter pointed to (mineralocorticoid,

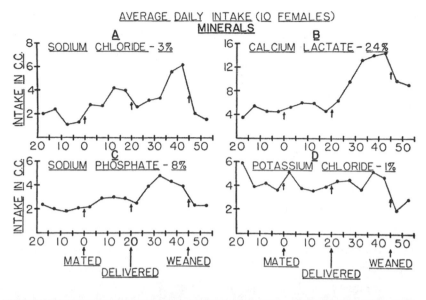

AVERAGE DAILY INTAKE (IO FEMALES)
MINERALS

A SODIUM CHLORIDE - 3%

B CALCIUM LACTATE - 24%

C SODIUM PHOSPHATE - 8%

D POTASSIUM CHLORIDE - 1%

MATED   DELIVERED   WEANED

MATED   DELIVERED   WEANED

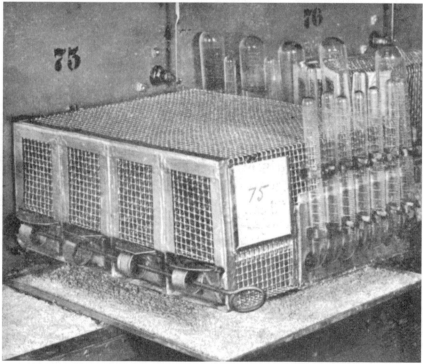

FIG. 3.4. *Top:* Ingestion of salts in pregnant and lactating rats. Note the increase in ingestion of sodium and calcium salts during pregnancy and lactation. *Bottom:* Self-selection cages. *Source:* Richter and Barelare 1938; Richter 1942–43

vitamin D, oxytocin, angiotensin), may also facilitate ingestive patterns (Denton 1982). In other words, hormones that conserve sodium, for example, can also participate in generating the behavioral responses of sodium ingestion (Denton 1982; Fitzsimons 1979).

PERSPECTIVE

Richter helped ignite the study of behavioral regulation of the internal milieu within the context of nutritional choice. There was little of this study within psychology itself, though this changed somewhat later when the phenomenon of taste aversion learning was discovered (see chapter 4). One area of study centered around the questions of which specific hungers were innate and which were learned, how many hungers there were, and how they were demonstrated.

Intellectually, Richter was mostly on the side of innate organization and therefore missed opportunities to investigate the interaction of innate predilection and learning. There were those (e.g., Harris et al. 1933) who argued that learning predominated in the food selections exhibited during the cafeteria experiments and the choosing of vitamin B by vitamin B–deficient rats. Others, like Richter, argued that dietary selection was an instinctive or innate predilection with variation in expression (Dove 1935). The innate conception and organization of behavior had, and still has, traction when the food choice is narrow (e.g., a choice between sodium or water), but when the choices are broad and the sensory signals are not succinct, learning must play a role (Rozin 1976b). This piece of psychobiology was outside of Richter's conceptual framework.

Nutrient search and identification are basic features of biological hardware. The laboratory rats Richter studied revealed several instances of specialized systems for water and sodium, calcium, perhaps phosphate ingestion, and perhaps some aspects of energy balance. The rats' solution was to approach a food source with caution, sample a small amount to determine the physiological outcome, and be wary of novelty (Rozin 1967, 1976b; see Chapter 4). Rats learning to avoid a food source that rendered them viscerally sick led to psychologists' recognition of long-delay learning, a process with rapid and profound lasting effects on behavior (Garcia, Hankins, and Rusiniak 1974; Rozin 1976b; see chapter 4). Visceral learning is a vital aspect of the mechanisms that operate during feeding. Determining what is making one sick is a vital piece of adaptation that requires distinguishing the novel from the familiar, learning what foods are safe, and limiting choices.

Long-delay learning is a real world event (Rozin and Kalat 1971; Garcia, Hankins, and Rusiniak 1974), and before the mid-1960s long-delay learning was not part of the intellectual arsenal of most behavioral psychologists. An important adaptation that Richter understood is the novel versus familiar dimension of food choice (see chapter 4). Amid the very general adaptive behavioral/physiological systems of the omnivorous rat are specialized systems for nutrient and mineral regulation of sodium, water, and calcium, for example (Rozin and Schulkin 1990).

Richter understood, as would many other investigators, that nutritional choice requires both specialized detector systems (Dethier 1976) and general forms of behavioral adaptation. When confronted with multiple choices, the vitamin-deficient rat may select one food source at a time and determine the outcome in terms of visceral effects (Rozin 1976b). Limiting choice, stabilizing outcomes, and determining consequences is a learning approach that no doubt operates in the success of self-selection.

As I have indicated, perhaps the extreme competence of the rats in Richter's self-selection experiments depended on the palatability of the choices (e.g., Kon 1931; Lat 1967; Galef 1991), how many choices there were, and in what manner the choices were offered (Tordoff 2002). This might explain the variability in replication of the self-selection experiments (e.g., Kon 1931; Harris et al. 1933; Lat 1967; Galef 1991).

Richter posited too many innate behaviors to explain the nutritional choice behaviors. There are limitations or constraints on both the successes and the failures of self-selection. The ability to self-select, when demonstrated, is perhaps less about evolutionary knowledge and more about the test conditions (Galef 1991).

Thus, one limitation of Richter's work was that learning played no role in the lexicon of scientific experimentation. The Psychobiology Laboratory emphasized the innateness of behavior. Another criticism is Richter's own failure to recognize the pervasive ways in which social learning facilitates food selection and avoidance (Galef 1991). Bennett Galef's experiments in a variety of contexts demonstrated that social cues, even for sodium sources, could facilitate food selection. Social context plays a part in alcohol consumption, something Richter studied, but he emphasized, perhaps naively, the adaptive role of alcohol in nutritional regulation.

MEYER, HOMEOSTASIS, ALCOHOL CONSUMPTION, AND NUTRITIONAL REGULATION

I now turn to the context in which Richter investigated homeostatic regulation and alcohol consumption. This line of research, which he began in the 1920s and continued until the 1950s, symbolized a number of interests for Richter. However, Adolf Meyer cautioned Richter that he felt the implications of Richter's research on alcohol might be misleading and worried that it might be misinterpreted and misused in what he referred to as the "alcohol controversies" (Meyer file of letters to Richter, Chesney Archives). Meyer was cautious; he did not want the research to be abused by the general public. It is instructive to look at this work at its outset.

The research began as a follow-up to Richter's dissertation work on spontaneous activity and both the internal and external signals that affect it (chapter 2). Richter did not invent the running wheel as a measure of rat activity, but he simplified and extended its use in the quantification of behavior. Nor was he the first to look at the effects of alcohol consumption on the running activity of the rat (Stewart 1898). Richter found that alcohol did influence spontaneous behaviors in rats (Richter 1926c). In a study that lasted several months, he offered each of several groups of rats, kept in different conditions, different concentrations of alcohol mixed with water. Six animals received 8 percent alcohol, twelve received 10 percent alcohol, and ten received 16 percent alcohol.

Richter noted that food consumption was related to the amount of alcohol ingested. His study suggested that growth patterns remained normal in the developing rats in which the experiments were done. The animals ate less food, however, depending on the concentration of alcohol they ingested. Alcohol, Richter hypothesized, was a source of energy. The animals regulated their energy intake by reducing the amount of regular food they ate (i.e., the McCollum diet) in proportion to the amount of alcohol they ingested.

Richter also conducted these experiments in mature rats and found a precise equilibrium of homeostatic energy. In a study with female rats, the caloric intake averaged over body weight was 167.87 kcal when ingesting 16 percent alcohol, 168.97 kcal when ingesting 10 percent alcohol, and 170.71 kcal when on the diet alone. The amount of food ingested reflected the amount of alcohol consumed, which resulted in homeostatic equilibrium across the three conditions.

Not many control subjects were used, and as usual no statistical analyses were done. Nevertheless, Richter demonstrated that total caloric intake was about the same for the female rats that consumed alcohol and those on the regular diet. He did the same for males, repeating this experiment several times and under different conditions.

Because he drew on both human and animal experiments wherever possible, Richter went on to look at taste psychophysics for alcohol in both rats and humans. The gustatory experiments were designed to characterize thresholds and to determine preferences for different concentrations of alcohol (Richter and Campbell 1940a). At what concentrations would alcohol be preferred over water? At what concentrations would it be clearly distinguishable from water?

In later years, Richter reported differences in rats' ingestion of different kinds of alcoholic beverages, such as wine and beer (Richter 1953). The focus again was on metabolic regulation, eating for calories. Approaching homeostatic regulation from the conceptual framework of a biological engineer, Richter concluded, "All the evidence at hand indicates that rats ingest only as many calories as they can utilize" (Richter 1953a, p. 536). He included the clinical message that "the modern user of alcoholic beverages should be made aware that he will probably do better by eating less food when he takes these beverages; that he will do best when he reduces his food intake in proportion to his caloric intake from the ingested alcohol" (Richter 1953a, p. 538).

Perhaps what made Meyer nervous about these experiments was the suggestion that alcohol could serve as a substitute for food in maintaining metabolic balance (Richter 1941a). Alcohol was seen as dangerous and a seduction. Richter's research was conducted in the conservative ambiance of Hopkins, the institution that ousted Watson for his sexual promiscuity, and under the ever-mindful watch of Meyer, who cautioned about how the results would be understood. Was alcohol a legitimate form of ingestive behavior to serve homeostatic behavior? Richter attempted to prove just that, linking this form of ingestive behavior to the homeostatic regulation of energy balance.

In a memorandum about the summary of Richter's alcohol article, Meyer stated, "I do not like to see contributions from the Clinic touching on questions of a problematic nature published without some safeguards of orientation as to the sense in which the contribution is offered" (Meyer files, Chesney Archives). A little later in the document he stated, "I am anxious to see that there is no temptation furnished to use the results of the study for unintended generalization by misquotation." Meyer was anxious that Richter state the limitations of his experiments at the outset. He had little quibble, in the letter, with the behavioral ingestive patterns and their role in metabolic regulation, but warned against getting embroiled in the "alcohol controversies." Interestingly, the paper, entitled "Alcohol as a Food" (Richter 1941a), would be one of the most often cited studies in the Richter corpus of research.

The range and approach of Richter's experimental sensibilities were expressed in these experiments, and despite the warnings of his mentor, Richter pursued this work. Later he would link thyroid activation to both running activity and alcoholic consumption. This research showed three emphases of Richter's work: (1) the fundamental role of biological clocks in behavioral and physiological regulation, (2) the regulation of the internal milieu, and (3) his comparative approach using animals and people.

Although Richter was not isolated, he worked alone. It is not clear what kind of input he received from colleagues. Richter, I think, did not have colleagues who critiqued his work and to whom he made himself vulnerable so much as he had important patrons of his work (G. Smith, pers. comm., November 2002). He assumed the validity of nutritional wisdom, seeing it as a piece of the hardware of bodily adaptation by which behavior serves regulatory physiology to promote viability. This was a prevalent cultural idea, one Richter breathed and assumed to be true. One significant scientist who was a major proponent of this view was Walter Cannon.

CANNON'S SUPPORT: THE NATIONAL RESEARCH COUNCIL

Cannon, as I indicated previously, was an early and important supporter of Richter's research. In correspondence between Cannon and Richter, Cannon alerted Richter to the fact that there are "considerable funds available for research in endocrinology" and asked whether Richter would join a committee of the National Research Council (Cannon Archives, Harvard University, March 16, 1936). This and other funding foundations had begun to play an important role in the rise of biomedical and other forms of research in the United States (Kohler 1991).

In another letter several months later, Cannon alerted Richter to a book on the appetitive behavior of sheep in South Africa (Harvard University Archives). Richter had found himself another patron, but had he found a colleague? Did he talk to Cannon about his experiments on gastric distention? That would have been difficult at that time, near the end of Cannon's life.

In fact, there was almost a decade (mid-1930s to mid-1940s) when Cannon was quite supportive of Richter's work, both in terms of intellectual encouragement and of financial support through the National Research Council, where Cannon chaired the Committee on Research in Endocrinology (see National Academy of Sciences Archives). Cannon was well aware of much of Richter's work on specific hungers and actively supported and promoted the research, as well as Richter's work on cycles. By 1944, however, the support from this source was diminishing. Cannon wrote to Richter, "Let me say personally that I regret that we have not felt justified in continuing our relations with your interesting work" (National Academy of Sciences Archives, April 25, 1944).

The National Research Council played an important role in supporting Richter's research project, and Cannon, sitting at its head, was well aware of Richter's latest findings and of his extension of the concept of homeostasis to a behavioral level of analysis. Cannon embraced Richter's behavioral findings with enthusiasm. They added a whole new dimension to the concept of homeostasis.

CONCLUSION

Richter understood the regulation of the internal milieu in the context of whole-body regulatory activity. He used the activity cage to monitor a broad array of rat behavior, including eating and drinking in the context of other regulatory activities, reflected in the active portion of their activity cycle (G. P. Smith 1997). Richter's contribution to the study of ingestive behavior is phenomenal; he provided real tools and biological explanations for regulatory events.

Richter clearly saw himself as building on the work of other investigators with regard to the selection of dietary requirements. From pigs (Evvard 1915) and rats (Osborne and Mendel 1918) to humans (Davis 1928), ideas about dietary self-selection of needed nutrients were in the intellectual air. "Dietary wisdom," a metaphor Cannon helped to popularize, was seen as a piece of our evolutionary legacy, experimentally expressed in a laboratory context.

Unfortunately, Richter had little intellectual room for the concept of learning and exaggerated the innate component in behavioral regulation of the internal milieu; innate engineering predominated his view of this behavioral adaptation. In this context, instinct means innate structure. Richter inherited this idea from his predecessors' study of self-selection. But there was no restraint placed on what the range of innate structures might be, and no real accounting for the failure of self-selection experiments by some investigators

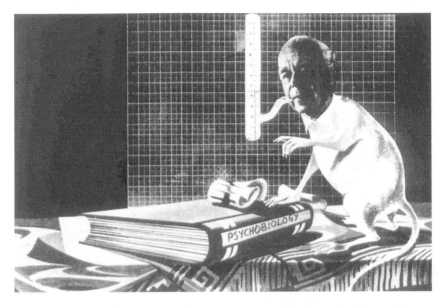

FIG. 3.5. Playful card depicting Richter ingesting something from what became known as a "Richter tube"

and the failure of animals to thrive when offered various choices in other experiments.

In his essay on the biology of drives, Richter argued that "the reason that human beings often make faulty dietary choices may be explained in part by parental guidance and advertisement" (1941c, p. 109). He suggested that "often when a child expresses a great appetite for certain substances, he is told by his parents that he must not eat them: equally often he is told to eat things which are very distasteful to him. He quickly learns to distrust his own appetite: and . . . comes under the influence of advertisements, he falls prey to them" (p. 109). The suggestion that culture degrades certain parts of our adaptive responses would be a recurrent theme in Richter's work. As noted in chapter 2, Richter mistakenly thought that circadian rhythms were lost in humans as a consequence of culture. Richter believed culture usually masked regulatory competence, although not always, as we will see in chapter 4.

Richter understood, as one commentator noted, "that the central problem for psychology was to discover the determinants of the initiation and termination of bouts of behavior" (Collier and Johnson 1997, p. 159). Richter did not think of behavior in modern ethological terms, in terms of a more modern cost-benefit analysis (Collier and Johnson 1997), or in ecological terms of the adaptation of species. Nor did he think much in terms of hedonic attraction (Young 1948), social learning (Galef and Whiskin 2001), or other forms of learning in the regulation of the internal milieu. What Richter did do was discover a rich assortment of behavioral and physiological forms of adaptation, suggest interesting routes for further inquiry, and remain close to his own data and the tradition of regulatory whole-body physiology.

Richter understood behavior as reflective of instinctive responses. Instinct was contrasted for years with intelligence and flexibility; then it was associated with the buildup of energy. Instincts were identified with drives, which could be satisfied through behavior—the hydraulic buildup and the depletion and repletion models. In this, Freud (1920/1975) was no different from Hull (1943) or many of the ethologists (Tinbergen 1951/1969); like other investigators of the time, he assumed some form of drive reduction for which behavior was pivotal to reduce excitation and arousal. This conception was common to various behavioral explanations.

Perhaps Richter understood instinct as Donald Hebb, Lashley's student, would: by asserting that "the problem of instinct is the correlative of that of intelligence, or insight, and of learning. It has just been seen that intelligence is not an entity that is quite distinct from learning and we may now see that instinct, also, is not to be cut off sharply from either" (Hebb 1949, p. 165). Instinct is about problem solving. We do not know Richter's views on this because he was not engaged at this level of scientific discourse. He assumed a concept like instinct and then set about demonstrating its validity.

How many innate or instinctive specific appetites are there? Certainly sodium is one, and perhaps calcium. Water seems a likely candidate, and protein remains a possibility. Avoidance of diets that render the animal ill, coupled with a tendency to be cautious of new nutritional options, seems to be operative in food choice, particularly for the omnivorous rat. The ecological adaptations are an essential part of discerning the range of strategies available for an animal to solve its nutritional requirements. Richter's work on nutritional selection was done largely using the rat, an omnivore with several noted specific appetites along with several more general behavioral strategies that serve it in the regulation of the internal milieu. Chapter 4 discusses further one strategy alluded to here, namely, learned taste aversion.

A playful sensibility abounded within the Richter laboratory; science was serious but fun business. Who but a whimsical person would produce a card like that in figure 3.5?

A Psychobiological Perspective on the Domesticated and the Wild

BIOLOGICAL AND CULTURAL CONTEXT

Richter was born in the century of Darwin's discoveries. Darwin often wrote about domestication and evolutionary change. During his first trip to the Galapagos Islands, as he recounted in *The Origin of Species,* Darwin was awed by the great variation in species (Darwin 1859/1965). His observations would eventually lead to his theory of natural selection and the idea that speciation developed through the selective pressures of geographical and ecological constraints. Ideas about adaptation, secondary sexual characteristic expression, and functional fit guided Darwin's thinking. To understand physiological and behavioral expression he looked to the niche, the organic conditions in which an animal had to live. In this adaptationist framework—an engineering, ecological context—Richter and many other students of animal behavior would feel very comfortable.

Darwin revolutionized the study of behavior by giving it a biological context. This was quickly adopted by those in the emerging field of psychology, and psychobiology was soon understood within the evolutionary context of adaptation. But Darwin held a Lamarckian perspective on certain hereditary changes, including use and disuse and intergenerational effects (S. J. Gould 2002). Use and disuse, instinct and habits, and the effects of domestication were dominant intellectual themes for Richter's predecessors and for Richter himself throughout his career; these categories figured in almost all of his investigations.

Darwin was worried by the price of domestication. He wanted "to estimate the amount of structural differences" that occurred as a result of cultural

imposition (Darwin 1859/1965, p. 38). The other concern that came to dominate his thinking was the inheritance component: instincts were seen as guid-
ing regulatory mechanisms in the organization of behavior. Richter was not
theoretical in general about the concept of instinct, but this concept was at the
root of his biological inquiry. The issue of biological predisposition, whether
rigid (as instinct was thought to be) or more malleable, was understood in
terms of behavioral and physiological adaptation. The Psychobiology Laboratory was centrally involved in this arena.

DOMESTICATION

In a number of his reviews on domestication, Richter pointed out that the rat
was an ideal animal to study. The animal was championed by Claude
Bernard's teacher, François Magendie (see also Holmes 1974, 2004) and, as I
have indicated, was introduced in this country as a laboratory animal by Adolf
Meyer in the early 1890s. Henry H. Donaldson expanded on the use of rats as
experimental subjects. Richter noted the experimental advantages of the rat,
including its diet, its similar physiology to humans, the ease with which it
reproduces under domestic conditions, its resistance to infection, and its
inclination toward domestication and resultant willingness to be handled.

One feature of rats noted early on was temperamental variance; some rats
were more aggressive than others. Yerkes, in a 1913 study, investigated the
heredity of savageness and wildness in rats. Within a few years, Richter would
be introduced to Yerkes at Harvard. Richter was greatly interested in measuring
the impact of experimental manipulations, not only on behavior but also on
physiology. The rat proved a convenient tool in this regard. Richter studied the
adrenal gland, among other end-organ systems, to observe the effects of domestication in the laboratory. The glandular structure of the inbred, domesticated
strains of rat differed from that of the wild hybrid, as did their less aggressive
nature (King and Donaldson 1929; King 1930). Darwin was right: domestication
altered both the internal physiology and the behavior of species.

Henry H. Donaldson was an important figure for Richter, as he had been for
Watson (Boakes 1984). Richter visited him often and knew him well. Donaldson, as noted earlier, was a teacher of Watson and the author of the book *The
Rat Data and Reference Tables for the Albino and the Norway Rat* (Donaldson
1915).[1] In this book, Donaldson described the "history of the rat since it
arrived in Western Europe" (Donaldson 1915, p. 111), the animals' life charts,
their behaviors, and the significant effects of domestication on their end-organ

systems, including the brain, which is smaller in the domesticated variant of rat. Interestingly, many decades later, enriched environments were shown to produce improvements in domesticated rats' neuronal structure and learning (Rosenzweig and Bennett 1996). Wild rats must be embedded in a much richer social context than domesticated rats.

EXPERIMENTAL CONTEXT

Before Richter and his colleagues embarked on their investigation, a body of evidence had already been gathered on the effects of domestication on rat behavior and physiology. For example, the adrenal gland had been demonstrated to be larger in the wild gray rat than in "the tame albino rat" (Donaldson 1915).

Richter's study revealed seasonal changes in the wild rats' adrenal size. Wild rats caught in the summer months had smaller adrenal glands than rats caught in the winter. Rogers and Richter (1948) noted that the effect was larger in males and that seasonal change in females was negligible (fig. 4.1). Of course, they gave only descriptive statistics (percentages, averages, etc.) in their paper, consistent with Richter's usual method. They mentioned seasonal differences only parenthetically, but did so with insight into the functional implications of size changes of the adrenal gland. Rogers and Richter (1948) cited conditions under which adrenal activities increased, including adaptation to colder temperatures and various forms of duress (Selye 1946). In addition to

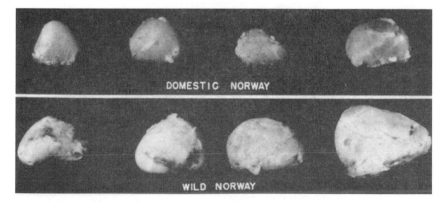

FIG. 4.1. Adrenal glands of the domestic and wild Norway rat. Note the apparent size difference in the wild and the domestic rat, matched by body weight of the animal. *Source:* Rogers and Richter 1948

several anatomical differences, they described the adrenal gland; the fasciculata and reticularis regions were thicker in undomesticated rats.

FAILURE TO EXPRESS THE BEHAVIORAL REGULATION OF SODIUM IN WILD RATS

Richter always returned to the phenomenon he took to be paradigmatic of a specific innate behavior: sodium ingestion following sodium loss or sodium need. For rats, domestication did have advantages, including the regulation of body sodium. Adrenalectomized domesticated rats, Richter discovered, survived quite well as long as they ingested sodium. Would wild rats also compensate for adrenalectomy and ingest sodium as a behavioral adaptation?

In a series of studies, Richter, Rogers, and Hall demonstrated that wild rat strains, captured in the streets of Baltimore, showed differences in sodium regulation from the domesticated variant. Both groups were adrenalectomized by the method that Richter had perfected in 1936 and 1941. As usual, both male and female rats were used. Using diets either rich or low in sodium, Richter and his colleagues looked at the regulation of sodium in food and in water. The rats always had water. Not surprisingly, both wild and domesticated strains died without access to sodium if the entire adrenal gland was removed (Richter, Rogers, and Hall 1950). Richter surmised that if partial tissue were left, the animals could survive without sodium, and he demonstrated that fact in the laboratory.

In experiments with what Richter called "salt therapy," he gave the rats a 3 percent NaCl solution. Richter noted a lot of variation in sodium intake in the wild strain of rat. The domesticated rats ingested the sodium more than the wild rats and had much higher survival rates. The study stated that the rate of survival was about 2 percent in the wild strain and 87 percent in the domestic strain (Richter, Rogers, and Hall 1950). Richter noted repeatedly that even the individual wild rats that increased their salt intake often died. This was not the case for the domestic variant.

Richter always emphasized "the high degree of suspiciousness of all new foods" in wild rats (Richter 1950c). Richter, Rogers, and Hall speculated that the wild rats' failure to increase their salt intake rested "chiefly on a psychological rather than a physiological basis" (1950, p. 239). They suggested that an exaggerated neophobia (suspicion of new food) in the wild strain impeded their regulatory competence in the confines of the safe laboratory. The wild rats died of a reluctance to sample and experience the beneficial effects of the sodium. Surprisingly, adjusting the concentration and forcing ingestion still resulted in fatality in the wild rats. Salt therapy, the researchers concluded, was not beneficial. To my knowledge, this experiment was never examined again. Subsequent studies have demonstrated both differences between strains and individual variation in sodium intake (e.g., Denton 1982; Roland and Fregly 1988).

Administering deoxycorticosterone to wild rats in addition to salt replacement still often resulted in death and in some instances caused sudden death. The wild variant was just less adaptive to changes in body sodium. Mosier and Richter reported that the adrenal glands of the domesticated rats were much more responsive to reductions in dietary salt concentration than were those of wild rats. On the low-sodium diet, the glomerulosa layer of the adrenal gland increased more in the domestic rat than in the wild rat (Mosier and Richter 1958). When placed on a high-sodium diet, both strains showed a reduction in adrenal size. Domestic rats increased their water intake to a greater extent than did wild rats. Of course, in both cases it is possible that changes could be observed more readily in domestic rats because their smaller baseline adrenal size made the effects of the switch to the low-sodium diet more noticeable. The wild rats, with their larger adrenal glands, presumably had more aldosterone and corticosterone in systemic circulation. Nonetheless, Mosier and Richter reported an anatomical difference in the domesticated and wild strains at the level of the zona glomerulosa (Mosier and Richter 1958).

That the wild variant did not demonstrate a sodium appetite in response to a sodium need, or to hormonal signals associated with sodium need, left many questions. Were the wild rats less adaptive than the domesticated rats? Was the experience of being trapped and transported traumatic, elevating levels of corticosterone enough to compromise wild rats' behaviors? What did this say about salt appetite, and was this phenomenon genetic or developmental? How long would a rat need to be domesticated to develop a salt appetite?

RATS, TASTE AVERSION, VISCERAL DISTRESS, AND POISONS

Richter's interest in self-selection paid off in his investigations of what rats ingest and what they avoid. He noted "in 1937, while studying the relation between the taste of substances and their nutritive or toxic values, I found that my laboratory rats have a remarkable ability to select nutritive substances and to avoid poisonous ones" (Richter 1948c, p. 255). Rats avoided certain kinds of tastes as if they could tell ingesting the substances would make them sick. For example, they avoided the toxin alpha-naphthylthiourea (ANTU). Richter studied this as part of his larger experimental interest in "bait shyness," the exaggerated neophobic response to possibly dangerous sources of foods or other objects.

GUSTATORY STUDIES: RATS AND PEOPLE

Richter designed psychophysical and taste avoidance tasks with several toxic substances. Building on his salt and sucrose psychophysical taste studies and comparing rats and people (Richter 1939a), he embarked on a study to determine taste thresholds for a number of toxic substances (Richter and Clisby 1941b). He knew that this taste had an innate genetic component, and he also wanted to contrast its study with previous studies of sucrose and salt taste. He presented human subjects with two glasses, one containing distilled water and the other containing the toxic compound. He wanted to determine the point at which the two substances could be distinguished. When subjects noted a definite bitter taste, this was considered the detection threshold.

Richter and Kathryn Clisby stated that "we know now that rats and human beings have almost identical taste thresholds for common sugar, salt, and phenylthiocarbamide" (Richter and Clisby 1941b, p. 163). This point can be disputed. Conducting the rat study, they added the toxic compound to a dextrose solution to facilitate its ingestion. Half the rats died within twelve hours, and the rest survived because they did not ingest significant amounts.

Some years later, Richter tested ten toxic compounds on basic gustatory psychophysical measures, using the same method that he had used earlier. He initially took the rats' rejection of toxic solutions to indicate a taste threshold. He saw their continued ingestion of both distilled water and a toxic compound as evidence that the rats had not reached their taste threshold for the toxin. Reduced ingestion indicated arrival at a threshold measure. But Richter also looked at what he called "a toxic symptom threshold," the concentration at which animals became sick (Richter 1950c).

The ten compounds included thallium sulfate, sodium fluoroacetate, thiosemicarbazide, arsenic trioxide, and ANTU. Richter noted that the gustatory properties of a toxic compound were linked to its solubility. Some of the toxins appeared to have no distinct taste, and he rightly asserted that a "tasteless toxic substance could not have existed widespread in nature in readily available forms at any time in evolutionary history, since in the absence of a taste warning every animal or man that ingested it would have perished" (Richter 1950c, p. 370). He noted that all of the tasteless compounds were not found in nature but made by humans. Though probably an exaggerated claim, this smacks of evolutionary common sense.

POISONING WILD RATS

In the 1940s, the U.S. military was interested in various kinds of poison warfare and thus supported Richter's research (Richter Archives, National Academy of Sciences). In collaboration with chemists from Dupont, Richter and his colleagues worked to generate a toxic substance that would be ingested by wild rats (Andrus et al. 1948).

First, though, he had to catch the rats. Richter and John Emlen modified a rabbit trap for use in capturing the wild rats of Baltimore, working with the city's Bureau of Street Cleaning.[2] The day before the traps were set, the areas where they were to be used were cleaned of debris. Using 265 traps, the researchers caught 70 rats on the first night and a total of 225 rats over a thirteen-day period for their initial study (Richter and Emlen 1945). Richter had noted in several places that, "owing to their high degree of suspiciousness, the wild rats are far more difficult to poison than are the domesticated rats" (Richter 1949a, p. 38).

In an interesting paper for the *Journal of the American Medical Association* on the incidence of rat bites, Richter wrote that "wild rats, even more than any domesticated animals, enjoy a very intimate living arrangement with man. They can live in the same house, share the same beds, eat the same foods, carry the same internal and external parasites, and suffer from the same diseases and plagues" (Richter 1945c, p. 324). He noted the incidence of rats biting people in Baltimore, specified where in the city the bites occurred, and even indicated what part of the body was bitten in each case (table 4.1).

Mentioning that the bites occurred while the victims were asleep and that twenty-some victims received multiple bites, Richter suggested that "a strong craving for blood might explain why, once having bitten a person, the rats apparently are apt to bite another." He then offered blood to several wild rats and noted that they ingested it. As always, Richter's interest in regulatory and cyclic phenomena and his medical focus (in this case, transmission of disease from rat to human) were at the heart of his research.

In a subsequent study on ANTU, Richter and his colleagues determined the effects of ANTU on pulmonary edema and changes in fluid balance in rats. They surmised that the toxic compound worked by causing pulmonary edema (a buildup of fluid in the lungs). They attempted to determine the extent to

TABLE 4.1. Parts of Body Bitten by Rats

Location	No. of Persons with Bites
Arms	
Hands and fingers	41
Forearm	5
Shoulder	2
Head	
Cheek, lips	11
Ear, eyebrow	5
Top of head	4
Legs	
Feet	19

Source: Richter 1945

which this occurred when rats were exposed to different amounts of the toxin (Dieke and Richter 1945; Richter and Emlen 1946; Richter 1952b). Richter was never squeamish experimentally, and in one study he bled rats to death so there would be no bleeding when their chests were opened.

Pulmonary edema began in the first hour after toxin ingestion. The lungs were full before the effusion of fluid into the pleural cavities. Lung weight was enhanced considerably by the administration of the toxic compound. Having observed pulmonary edema in these animals, Richter documented other physiological changes, including immunological changes. He concluded that the toxic poisoning shifted large amounts of extracellular fluid to the lungs. Later he would report species variation in this response (Dieke and Richter 1945; unpublished results cited in Dieke and Richter 1946a).

In one study, Sally Dieke and Richter looked at variation in rats' responses to poison across strain, age, and gender. They injected ANTU intraperitoneally or administered it by intragastric intubation, varying the dose by body weight. They found fewer fatalities in the youngest rats. Suckling rats and young rats weighing less than 200 grams were six times more resistant to the poisoning. They reported no difference with gender (Dieke and Richter 1946a).

Richter also noted that removal of various endocrine tissues—the thyroid, parathyroid, and gonads—did not alter the rats' response to the toxin. He thought that perhaps the weight of a rat's adrenal glands might contribute to its vulnerability to toxicity. In other experiments, he mixed different amounts of the toxin into the stock McCollum diet and gave the rats water ad libitum (Richter 1946a). He wanted to determine the rats' tolerance of and survival rates after ingestion or noningestion of the diet.

Richter was also interested in further determining the gustatory and visceral mechanisms of the tongue and other organs of the alimentary tract that may contribute to the vulnerability of domestic and wild rats to toxins. Richter and his colleagues first determined the structure of the tongue of the domestic rat (Fish, Malone, and Richter 1944) and then expanded their investigations to the wild rat (Fish and Richter 1946). They noted that the tongue of the domestic rat was smaller than that of the wild rat by about 17 percent. In another study, Richter and Emmett Hall looked at intestinal length in wild and domestic rats and found that the wild rats had longer intestines, which they speculated contributed to the differences in vulnerability to the toxins (Richter and Hall 1947).

Richter described some unique characteristics of the wild rats in context of these poisoning experiments. These included what he described as "psychotic behavior," which he speculated was induced by an exaggerated fear of food poisoning. Richter summarized the core finding of the poisoning experiments as follows: if the rats survived the poisoning, they learned to avoid the food source. He also described the doses that resulted in avoidance or fatality: the concentration at which rats learned food avoidance was within a small range of 0.03 to 0.09 percent; doses higher than this killed rats straight away, and lower doses did not make them ill at first exposure. Those wild Norway rats that became ill but survived the poisoning, however, displayed what Richter described as "psychotic" behavior (though just "bizarre" might have been more accurate). The rat, during both the light and dark periods, would hold itself erect at the back of the cage, standing on its hind legs and holding onto the top of the cage (fig. 4.2). One of Richter's assistants called the phenomenon "straphanging." Richter then noted that "often one foot was held in the air in a manner reminiscent of the postures seen in catatonic patients." The normally escape-prone wild rats remained frozen in this posture. Richter inferred that the poisoning experiences induced "abnormal" behaviors (Richter 1950b).

BAIT SHYNESS

The self-described "reluctant rat-catcher" (Richter 1968b) caught many rats in the wilds of Baltimore city over a ten-year period. He tackled this part of his research, which consisted of scanning a rough environment for wild rats on which to test modern substances that might be linked to genetic taste functions. The landscape of alleys and yards was a long way away from his Colorado youth, but, drawn to the Norway rat and its study, Richter quickly

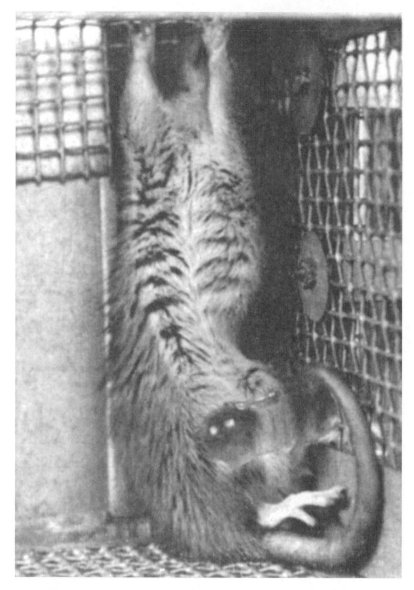

FIG. 4.2. Abnormal prolonged "straphanging" posture of a rat exposed to a toxic compound. *Source:* Richter 1950b

became fascinated by the whole phenomenon. Chasing down the rats was almost an urban version of his early hunting days in Colorado.[3]

Of course, bait shyness and the difficulty of poisoning rats had been known for ages and documented in several investigations, including Richter's. Wild rats' reluctance to ingest unfamiliar foods is a special behavioral adaptation that serves them well in tagging food sources and, most importantly, in linking specific food ingestion with visceral distress in animals in which taste and olfaction are essentially tied to food regulation (Rozin 1976b; Garcia, Hankins, and Rusiniak 1974).

Richter was close to suggesting something like a form of taste aversion with his emphasis on "bait shyness," food avoidance, and visceral distress from poisoning. Noticing the relationship between the concentrations of toxins and rats' avoidance of them, he found that rats stopped eating poisoned food after it "made them sick" (Richter 1946a, p. 366) (fig. 4.3). Richter acknowledged that the mechanism of this response "has not been determined. It could depend on association of ill effects with the taste of ANTU or smell" (Richter 1946a, p. 370).

Of course, being close and nailing it are quite different. Richter was also looking at the development of tolerance to toxins by small exposures to them. Perhaps he missed the boat on taste aversion learning because he ignored the learning part of behavior, remaining instead outside the intellectual battles of psychology.

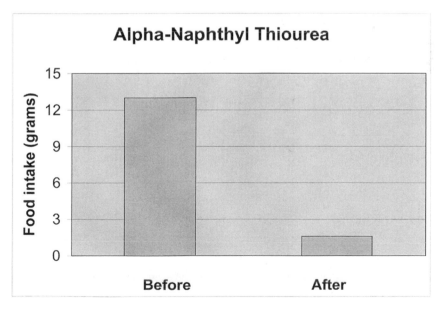

FIG. 4.3. Ingestion of food sources before and after exposure to a toxic compound. *Source:* Data from Richter 1946a

Taste aversion learning became a special case: a very specific biological form of learning (Garcia, Hankins, and Rusiniak 1974). A variety of animals associated the ingestion of a food source with visceral illness. This is a specialized form of learning outside of the immediate realm of associative learning (see Rozin 1976b). The learning of an association can take hours; there are constraints on learning because stimuli are not all equal in their associative potential. For Richter's rats, gustatory stimuli took precedence over visual stimuli; the converse held for birds, in which visual acuity is more evolved than it is in rats (Shettleworth 1972; Rozin 1976b).

Richter did not lose track of real-world events such as light/dark cycles, thirst, fear, and food ingestion the way many psychologists in North America tended to during the dominance of learning theory across academic psychology.[4] Richter probably understood bait shyness, what later became known as "taste aversion learning," in terms of adaptive specialization. Of course, if he had been more oriented toward a theoretical approach that included learning, he might have discovered that some stimuli were more closely linked to gastric distress than others.

Richter continued to write and think about his experiments and experiences as a "reluctant rat-catcher" for some time after the work in the late 1930s and 1940s. In a late article (Richter 1968b), he described the poisoning experiments, catching wild rats, being bitten, and his respect for this hardy animal. At the time of this publication, the work on taste aversion was about to be understood within psychology and psychobiology. The article makes no mention of the emerging work on taste aversion learning. This work would have a profound effect on psychology (Rozin and Kalat 1971; Garcia, Hankins, and Rusiniak 1974).

TEMPERAMENTAL FEATURES OF THE WILD
AND THE DOMESTICATED RAT

Though bait shyness is part of the normal wariness of most wild rats (e.g., Barnett 1956, 1963), social wariness is sometimes linked to temperament; in groups of rats, some individuals are more wary of unusual objects than are others (e.g., Hall 1941).

Darwin described shyness as behavior toward something socially unfamiliar (Darwin 1872/1998). But evidence of strain and individual differences pervades the animal literature, which recognizes an animal's temperament as a factor in shyness. Differences between individuals of a species reflect temperamental characteristics, for example, the degree of reluctance to sample a food source or of aggression or tameness. Individual differences are also often linked to differences in problem-solving abilities.

Fear of unfamiliar objects is a basic, broad-based biological predisposition for a wide range of animals, including humans (Hebb 1949; Kagan 1989). This fear has long been noted by investigators (Sadovnikova-Koltzova 1926) and was central to Richter's work on bait shyness, strain differences, and the effects of domestication. But some animals are, by their biological predisposition, more or less likely to approach or avoid a food source.

Richter had found it much easier to poison domesticated rats than their wild counterparts, and had concluded that the price of civilization is the reduction of biological wariness of new, unfamiliar objects. But we still do not know what role temperament played in the poisoning experiment. What if the particular group of wild rats Richter caught happened to be unusually shy, or his group of domesticated rats was especially unwary by temperament? If domestication is a factor in wariness, how long do rats have to be domesticated before they become less wary?

HOPELESSNESS AND VOODOO DEATH

Richter was always intellectually close to Cannon. Both scientists were rooted in regulatory physiology and the maintenance of bodily viability. Cannon, in an influential though speculative paper for *American Anthropologist,* theorized that individuals frightened to despair were vulnerable to "sudden death" (Cannon 1942). Superstitious fear was linked to this sudden death—sometimes called voodoo death. In what were commonly referred to at that time as "primitive" cultures, voodoo death occurred when a person was literally frightened to death by an experience imposed on him or her by a shaman or other individual.

Cannon had long been interested in what William James called "the energies of men" (James 1907/1968), the range of energy required to sustain action (Benison, Barger, and Wolfe 1987). As Benison, Barger, and Wolfe noted, "Cannon found the idea [of voodoo death] provocative and at once took steps to exploit its similarities to some of his own experimental observations" (Benison, Barger, and Wolfe, 1987, pp. 316–17). Cannon believed a feeling of hopelessness was endemic to the state preceding voodoo death and rendered an individual vulnerable to pathology and the breakdown of bodily adaptation and the energies of humans.

Referring to anecdotal evidence of human voodoo death, Cannon asked whether "those who have testified to the reality of voodoo death have exercised good critical judgment" (Cannon 1942, p. 171). He cited William James's comments on the profound vulnerability of socially isolated individuals, cut off from their peers and their community, to voodoo death. Voodoo death often occurred in individuals who were ostracized from the community. Noting that persistent fear without relief can cause a harmful chronic activation of the sympathetic and adrenal systems, Cannon concluded that "voodoo death may be real, that it may be explained as due to shocking emotional stress" (Cannon 1942, p. 180).

In his essay on sudden death, Richter picked up the Cannon theme of a "state of shock" and then went on to state that "as so often happens, this phenomenon was discovered during the course of other experiments" (Richter 1957f, p. 193). Richter and his colleague Gordon Kennedy were studying sodium metabolism and trimmed rats' whiskers so that sodium trapped on them would not contaminate other food sources. Richter then moved on to an experiment in which he measured endurance and survival times of domesticated and wild rats forced to swim in water. This was somewhat analogous to survival times after prolonged ingestion of only one nutrient (fat, protein, etc.). He began the studies with domesticated rats. Richter observed that survival time was related to water temperature. Of interest was that "at all temperatures a small number of rats died within 5–10 minutes after immersion." Then emerged a Richter moment: "Would a rat swimming without whiskers show the peculiar behavior of the rat in the metabolism cage?" (Richter 1957f, p. 194). He observed that about one-third of the twelve domesticated rats with clipped whiskers that he tested died rapidly.

Richter then turned his attention to hybrid wild and domesticated rats, and found that five of the six hybrid rats died within a brief five- to ten-minute period. When Richter looked at the effects of clipped whiskers on wild rats, he found that all thirty-four of the wild rats with clipped whiskers died rapidly when placed in the water. Richter noted that these rats were newly trapped and that, as part of the whisker-cutting procedure, the rats had been transported in a black bag from a holding facility. The rats had been immobilized for a time because, as Richter noted, "held in this way, the rats can neither bite nor escape" (1957f, p. 196).

Richter concluded that the wild rats had lost "all hope of escape." He observed that some of the wild rats died simply from being held in the black bag. Richter noted that the situation was "one of hopelessness: whether they are restrained in the hand or confined in the swimming jar, the rats are in a situation against which they have no defense. This reaction of hopelessness is shown by some wild rats very soon after being grasped in the hand and prevented from moving: they seem literally to give up" (Richter 1957f). Richter noted that the wild rats were more susceptible to this sudden death. So, while whisker clipping was incidental to avoiding food contamination and animal restraint was incidental to whisker clipping, it appeared that perhaps both of these events were instrumental in provoking hopelessness and even death.

A phenomenon called "learned helplessness" (Seligman 1972) would be understood sometime later and would become an important part of academic psychology. In one example of learned helplessness, rats and dogs were placed in an uncontrollable aversive context; they were unable to avoid electric shock. When later given an opportunity to avoid the shock, they were less likely to do so as a function of the prior experience. They had presumably learned that their avoidance behaviors were ineffective, and they tended to give up.

Some of Richter's results, though not all, were replicated by other investigators (cf. Grifiths 1960; Hughes and Lynch 1978). Hughes and Lynch noted that hopelessness might not be the best explanation; it was still not clear why the wild rats tended to drown to a much greater degree than did the domesticated rats after their vibrissae had been shaved and they had been held for a period of time. The reasons for this reaction, which was particularly common in wild rats, remain unexplained (Boice 1973; Hughes and Lynch 1978). Hughes and Lynch could only conclude that wild rats were much more vulnerable to drowning than the domestic rats (Hughes and Lynch 1978).

Neil Miller, the experimental psychologist, commented, "If you give these rats a chance to escape just once from this situation, when you later expose them again they will keep swimming for a long time" (Miller 1979, p. 44). But this concept of learning and expectation was not the sort of thing that Richter would go after with experimental gusto.

What Richter observed in the wild rat was a failure of behavioral adaptation. In the wild, a physiological response to an external event leads to a behavioral response, such as flight or biting, which in turn leads quickly to either success or failure. In the laboratory, however, such behavior was prevented. Adaptation was degraded, making the wild rats more vulnerable to a broad array of behavioral failures.

THE PROBLEM OF DOMESTICATION: BACK TO CANNON

Richter depicted voodoo death as not just a feature of "primitive" cultures, describing instances in our culture of deaths from excessive fear in war. Richter observed, "A phenomenon of sudden death has been described that occurs in man, rats, and many other animals, apparently as a result of hopelessness: this seems to involve overactivity primarily of the parasympathetic systems. In this instance as in many others, the ideas of Walter Cannon opened up a new area of interesting, exciting research" (Richter 1957f; Blass 1976, p. 329). Wolfe, Barger, and Benison recognized Richter's relationship to Cannon's work, commenting that "fifteen years later 'voodoo death' was reprinted in an issue of *Psychosomatic Medicine* that contained papers presented at a meeting of the American Psychosomatic Society held in 1957 to memorialize Cannon. Among the contributions was one by Curt P. Richter of Johns Hopkins, which followed up Cannon's article" (Wolfe, Barger, and Benison 2000, p. 479).

W. H. Gantt, Richter's colleague at the Phipps Clinic at Hopkins and translator and disciple of Pavlov, held a conference celebrating the twenty-fifth anniversary of the Pavlovian Laboratory at Hopkins. The proceedings of the conference were published as a book, *Physiological Bases of Psychiatry* (Richter 1958e).

In his presentation at this conference, Richter made no mention of Pavlov. The research he discussed was rooted not in Pavlov but in Cannon (Richter 1958e). Richter noted that it was Philip Bard, his colleague at Hopkins and a student of Cannon, who called his attention to the phenomenon of sudden death. He commented that "the reading of Cannon's paper stimulated me to start a search on a wider basis for an explanation of the sudden unexplained death in our rats. This search has led me to many new and unexplained fields" (Richter 1958e, p. 117).

Extending what I described above, Richter made the point that he noticed sudden death primarily in the wild rats, which he knew had larger adrenal glands. The rat felt trapped and unable to cope or to remove itself from the aversive situation. In Richter's own research, when rats were forced to swim for a long period, few of the rats that were not held died, whereas many of those that were held died. In other words, when Richter held rats for a period of time, he noted, "such a reaction of apparent hopelessness is shown by some wild rats very soon after being grasped in the hand and prevented from moving. They seemed literally to give up" (Richter 1958, p. 120).

DOMESTICATION, SCIENCE, AND CIVILIZATION

Richter extended experimentally Darwin's concept of domestication, which had been discussed in the literature for more than fifty years (e.g., Yerkes 1913), applying his laboratory state of mind to the problem. He noted that since the publication of Darwin's book on domestication (Darwin 1868/1892), one species—the Norway rat—had been domesticated for a specific purpose (Richter 1949b). This animal was used "not as a source of food or clothing, not as a pet, but as an animal for scientific research in all branches of biology and medicine" (Richter 1949b, p. 379).

Darwin noted that "in all parts of the world, man has subjected many animals and plants to domestication or culture" (1868/1892, 1:2). He also observed the morphological effects of domestication in a wide variety of species. This was the background against which Richter embarked on his own studies on domestication. Some systems, such as reproduction, were enhanced by domestication. In Darwin's words, "our domesticated animals, which have been long habituated to a regular and copious supply of food, without the labor of searching for it, are more fertile than corresponding wild animals. It is notorious how frequently cats and dogs breed, and how many young they produce at birth" (Darwin 1868/1892, 2:89).

Of human evolution, Richter wrote that "primitive man lived in an environment in which physical strength, endurance and aggressiveness were at a premium" (Richter 1952a, p. 273). He said about what he assumed was the "growth of community life" that the more aggressive forms of behavior of the "primitive state" became less important as civilization developed (p. 273). Of course, this explanation of our behavioral biology is now outdated; we know that cooperation, deception, and cunning were just as important to our biological legacy as overt aggressiveness.

Richter asserted that "the wild Norway rat, like primitive man, lives in an environment in which it must constantly be on the alert and often has to fight for its very existence" (Richter 1952a, p. 275). Of course, we modern humans also fight for existence, and perhaps the reduction of adrenal capacity (assuming a phenomenon observed in animals whose food options are less predictable and less easily accessible also applies to us) is an important adaptation as we shift our metabolic and cognitive resources elsewhere. Richter, following his intellectual predecessor Cannon, focused on the adrenals because of their vital function in adapting to duress.

Richter, always mining his data, recalled that spontaneous running occurred less in domesticated rats than in wild rats. Fasting produced much greater activity in wild rats than in domestic rats (Richter and Rice 1954). Richter and Uhlenhuth noted that no such difference in running activity was found in the wild variant when compared with the domestic variant after gonadectomy. The article suggests that the reduction in adrenal gland activation is compensated for by a greater dependence on gonadal secretion. This is nice evolutionary physiology hand waving. The reasons for the larger pituitary gland in the domestic strain of rat began to look confusing, and Richter acknowledged some of the confusion but did not really engage the issue. He used biology just enough to open discussion (table 4.2).

In "Domestication of the Norway Rat and Its Implications for the Problem of Stress," Richter asserted that "the use of the captive wild rat" represented "the completely wild animal in its free state" (Richter 1949a, p. 42). He also suggested that cultural selection tended to favor the tamer rats, the ones that were more easily handled by humans. Richter then suggested that "the diseases of adaptation" (Selye 1946) were a feature of domestication. Richter focused in these studies on how the effects of civilization both aid us (increasing our ability to solve problems of self-selection) and diminish our physiology (making our adrenal glands less robust).

TABLE 4.2. Comparison of Weights of Organs of
Domestic and Wild Norway Rats

Larger in Wild Norway Rats	Larger in Domestic Norway Rats	Same Size
Adrenals	Pituitary	Lungs
Brain	Thymus	Ovaries
Heart	Uterus	Testes
Kidney		
Liver		
Pancreas		
Preputials		
Prostate		
Seminal vesicles		
Spleen		
Thyroid		

Source: Richter 1949b

As Richter understood it, the effects of domestication interacted with an individual's temperament and personal features, and particularly with individual variation of activity and inactivity (see also Kagan 1989). Richter suggested that some individuals had "richer" systems and expressed more "pep" (Richter 1932). He saw clock mechanisms at work in activity and inactivity (Richter 1932).

CONCLUSION

Richter's roving experimental eye brought him to taste aversion learning, a phenomenon that would later have a profound effect on American psychology and the understanding of learning. Richter, rooted in biological considerations, simply understood that a normal reluctance to ingest unfamiliar foods made wild rats difficult to trap, and that gustation was a primary sensory modality and part of the alimentary canal that included gastrointestinal functions. This phenomenon would play an important role in the coming battles about the biological basis of learning. But the ideological battles were not Richter's concern. It was the phenomenon itself that interested him.

Richter inherited the problem of domestication's influence on behavior and physiology and certainly made important contributions to this area of inquiry. The effects of domestication on a variety of behavioral and end-organ systems are now fairly well known (e.g., Price 1984, 2002).

Richter always maintained a practical, clinical focus on the effects of domestication by culture. A good deal of this research was done during World War II and was supported because of a prevailing emphasis on what was called military research, or military medicine. Richter suggested that the study of the wild rat could help in the war effort (Study of Wild Rats, Richter Archives, National Academy of Sciences).

The Committee on Medical Research supported Richter's research on bait shyness and food aversion learning, the ANTU ingestion research (Ormsbee 1948). In an article written for *Advances in Military Medicine,* Ormsbee cited Richter's work on "rodent control," describing how "ANTU was shown to be a valuable weapon in the control of the common Norway rat" (Ormsbee 1948, p. 654). Richter housed his research in real-world events; practical implications were always in close proximity.

Richter assumed a whole set of cultural ideas, some of which emerged from biology, others from the social sciences. He never argued for his ideas; he made assumptions and then sought their demonstration. He invented instruments, developed experimental methods, and examined data. Richter began his investigations with an adaptationist conception of evolution (see S. J. Gould 2002 for limitations of this view) and the use and disuse of morphological and behavioral expression.

Richter expanded on a problem of domestication that began with Darwin. Both the work of Donaldson on domestication and the speculations of Cannon on voodoo death figured importantly in Richter's investigations. Richter mentioned that he visited Donaldson often (Richter 1985); one assumes this was to discuss the interesting findings Richter discovered in his laboratory.

Richter was one of a number of individuals looking at the effects of domestication on end-organ systems (King and Donaldson 1929), work that would continue over a long period (e.g., Price 2002). Domestication and temperament influence a wide variety of behavioral and physiological events, including rats' activity patterns and escape behaviors (Price 2002), and Richter's work fits nicely within a tradition of exploring these phenomena.

Richter referred to "captive wild rats as validly representing the completely wild animal in its free state" (Richter 1949a, p. 42). But what is a free state? Typically it is conceived of as the opportunity to succeed or fail in the attempt to survive and reproduce. In Richter's rats, the effects of domestication were reduced suspiciousness and ferocity due to lower levels of adrenal secretion, but better reproductive ability due to larger gonads. If Richter was entirely consistent he would have noted that domestication had great benefit, namely reproductive fitness. In other words, perhaps one advantage of domestication was an ability to easily express a sodium appetite (and a corresponding increase in longevity) and a greater ability to reproduce, thanks to higher levels of estrogen and lower levels of cortisol. These events, Richter suggested, parallel our own evolution, in which better adjusted but physically weaker individuals emerged: us moderns. Richter wondered whether the "diseases of adaptation" Hans Selye (1946) described (e.g., adrenal atrophy) were a reflection of domestication, writing, "In summary, the experiment started 100 years ago with the domestication of the Norway rat may help throw some light on trends of development of animals that live in a controlled environment and of the factors involved in the production of these trends. It may also give us data that will help to study the effects that the controlling of the environment may have had on man" (Richter 1949a, p. 45).

In a commentary at the end of this article, Selye noted, "I have followed Dr. Richter's work for many years and I so heartily agree with his conclusions

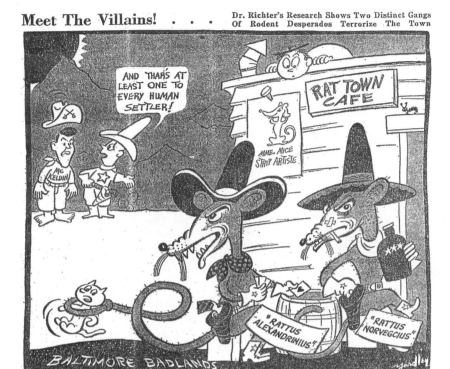

FIG. 4.4. Cartoon about Richter's work which appeared in a Baltimore newspaper. *Source:* © 1944, the *Baltimore Sun*. Reprinted with permission.

that I think I am the wrong man to discuss the paper. I feel that the interpretation of his data which he has given is very well supported" (Selye 1946, p. 45).

Richter noted three types of selection: selection in the wild, cultural selection by humans in an uncontrolled environment, and selection in a "controlled environment" (Richter 1949a, p. 45). This version of social Darwinism sought to explain the "production of the so-called weaker, the milder, better-adjusted individual" (Richter 1952a, p. 283). Richter wrote that the human "resembles . . . our domesticated Norway rat—happily living out its caged existence" (Richter 1952a, p. 283). This is a long way from the freedom of Colorado and the West where Richter grew up. He was clearly worried about the effects of domestication and the controlled environment on human physiology and human heredities.

A glorified conception of freedom and our restrained wild nature guided Richter (1953f) and manifested itself in this inquiry, as well as in his suspicion of what he called "designed research." He was wary of the consequences of the controlled environment on human freedom, expression, and physiology. Of course, this notion is romantic, seductive, and can be misguided.

It is not clear to what extent Richter understood the possible limitations of the work and of his point of view. He was best at embarking on interesting empirical investigations. Though the details or the mechanisms remain unclear, the science was, I submit, endlessly interesting.

Richter's work did not go unnoticed by the local newspaper in Baltimore (fig. 4.4).

CHAPTER 5

Neurobiological Investigations and Clinical Applications

LESSONS LEARNED IN PANAMA

As noted in previous chapters, Curt Richter's orientation to the brain and the organization of behavior was influenced greatly by Adolf Meyer, a neurologist by training and a student of the great nineteenth-century neurologist Hughlings Jackson (1884/1958). Jackson, among others, suggested that the evolution of the brain mirrored the evolution of a species: the more advanced the species, the more corticalized the brain; the dissolution of the nervous system was the breakdown of function, the converse of the evolutionary trend (Critchley and Critchley 1998).

Richter was interested in behavioral adaptation, the idea that, as James put it, "all nervous centers have then in the first instance one essential function, that of intelligent action" (James 1890/1952, p. 79). Predominant in this view was that the organization of action was dependent on the forebrain and that the basic reflexes were mediated by the brain stem. This theme in neurological research today remains a viable hypothesis about the organization of behavior and the levels of neural integration (Grill and Norgren 1978). As Richter began his studies on the sloth during his trip to Panama, neurological inquiry would play a fundamental role, as would the idea of levels of neural function. These would remain important aspects of Richter's research throughout his career.

Two Hopkins figures, Meyer and Watson, influenced Richter's travel to and work in Panama. Meyer provided the resources for Richter to travel to that country to study the neurological basis of behavior. The grasp reflex Richter would focus on there was of paramount importance to Watson (1919; see Boakes 1984), and Richter inherited this interest.

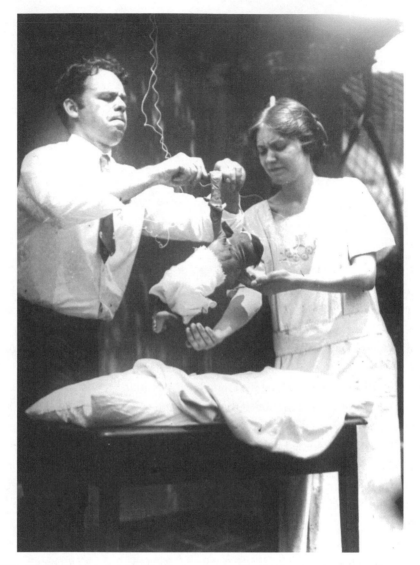

FIG. 5.1. Newborn infant hanging from apparatus designed to test the grasp reflex. *Source:* Richter 1934c

The grasp reflex had already been identified in newborns. Watson described this phenomenon in print and in his promotional films about behaviorism and reflexes. Richter wrote, "I have attempted to carry this work a step farther along the line of Watson's original experiments: first by putting it on an objective basis, with a method for measuring the strength of the reflex" (Richter 1934c, p. 327). Note the comment about the contrast to Watson—an "objective basis."

Richter began this exploration with a set of experimental objectives that he would continue to pursue throughout his career. They were (1) to study the grasp reflex from a distinctively neurological and physiological orientation, (2) to measure skin resistance (a clinical technique that he inherited from Meyer), and (3) to investigate broad-based neurological phenomena by combining neurological, behavioral, and clinical scientific perspectives. Richter always had an eye toward the patient; because he worked in a hospital clinic, his experiments had clinical applications. His neurological investigations were perhaps most important clinically.

TROPICAL FORESTS IN PANAMA

The Panama Canal was completed in 1914. Its building necessitated the deliberate flooding of areas of tropical forest. The high ground of Barro Colorado ("Red Clay") Island came into being due to that flooding. By 1923, the island had become a research bastion for a number of scientists, a small tropical forest rich with animal life. One major figure at the newly formed island was the naturalist Thomas Barbour (1943), who helped shape it into a research institute (Leigh 1999).

Barro Colorado research station was originally funded by foundations and universities, under the direction of the National Research Council, to foster biological research. It has now become part of the Smithsonian Tropical Research Institute. The island is home to many mammalian species, birds, reptiles, and amphibians (see Leigh 1999) (fig. 5.2).

A report by Thomas Barbour, chair of the Executive Committee for the Institute for Research in Tropical America, identified Adolf Meyer as the sponsor of Richter's sojourn to the research island. The Johns Hopkins University (at Meyer's suggestion) contributed $300. Richter was listed in notes on the island's visitations as follows: "Dr Curt Richter, Johns Hopkins Medical School, Baltimore, MD, experimental physiologist: studied the sloth principally, but used monkeys and some other mammals as well. Plan to return with two associates to continue research next summer" (Annual Report of the Barro Colorado Island Biological Station, March 7, 1925). Judging by the descriptions, either conditions were minimal or Richter was very frugal: an entry dated August 8 lists $30.35 spent on "subsistence," and one dated September 16 lists $16.65 for subsistence and $1.20 for supplies.

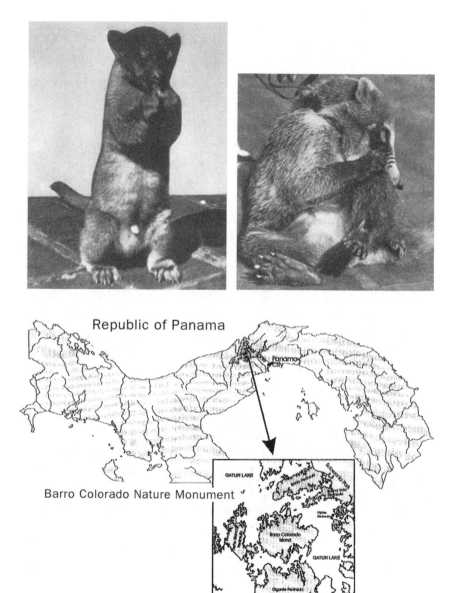

FIG. 5.2. *Top:* Two of the animals Richter worked with on his sojourn to Panama: *left,* a coatimundi; *right,* a kinkajou. *Bottom:* A map of Barro Colorado. *Source:* Richter 1925; Barro Colorado, Republic of Panama

For Richter's second and final trip to the Institute, the visitation log reads, "Dr Curt P. Richter, Johns Hopkins Hospital, Baltimore, MD, continued his studies begun at the island last year in experimental physiology using as subjects the sloths and monkeys" (Annual Report of the Barro Colorado Island Biological Station, March 7, 1925).

Richter's trips to Panama were rare sojourns into a naturalistic paradise for a scientist rooted in the laboratory. One of the papers he published based on those excursions was entitled "Some Observations of the Self-Stimulation Habits of Young Wild Animals" (Richter 1925). Richter noted how human self-stimulation, "thumb and finger sucking and erotic habits," would serve our understanding "from a more biological point of view" (Blass 1976, p. 148). The following are his anecdotal observations.

Richter began the article by noting that "during the past summer in Panama I had opportunity to make a few observations on several forms of self-stimulation habits of three wild animals: a coatimundi, a kinkajou, and a spider monkey" (Blass 1976, p. 148). He observed the behavior of a young female coatimundi on a colleague's patio. He noted that the animal had a habit of sucking and chewing on her knee. This was a common occurrence, but when given other behavioral options, the animal ceased this behavior.

The second animal Richter observed, a young male kinkajou, had been raised by a physician. The kinkajou had a habit of "autofellatio so firmly fixed that the physician was unable to break it" (Blass 1976, p. 150).

A spider monkey was the third subject of his observations. It, too, was raised in the home of a colleague, who took it in after its mother was shot. It was treated as a member of the family, eating and sleeping with other family members. Richter observed that the monkey sucked its finger and displayed childlike behaviors.

Richter noted in the same paper that "in all three animals the self-stimulation activity was suckling" (Blass 1976, p. 151). Richter speculated that the suckling behavior originated in utero, was a source of comfort throughout the animals' development, and was expressed in a variety of mammals. In making this observation, he was neither observing nor reporting on the animal in the wild terrain of Panama. Instead, the animals were observed on front porches.

Richter's behavioral observations were in line with the earlier approaches to developmental observation reported by Lashley and Watson (1913), who described one or more animals over a period of weeks. Their work too was supported by Meyer.

BEHAVIORAL/NEUROLOGICAL STUDIES

STUDIES ON THE GRASP REFLEX

Richter's major study in Panama was a neurological examination of the effects of decerebration in the sloth on sensory motor rigidity (Richter and Bartemeier 1926).

Richter would acknowledge in his paper on the sloth:

> The experimental part of this work was done by Dr. Richter, with the aid and suggestions of Dr. George B. Wislocki, in Panama at the Institute for Research in Tropical America. Dr. Richter wishes to express his indebtedness to the Institute for the assistance and facilities offered for carrying on this and other work during the summer months of 1924 and 1925. Thanks are due especially to Mr. James Zetek, custodian of the laboratory, and to Dr. Ignanzio Molino, assistant custodian, for their tireless efforts in helping to procure the necessary materials and animals. The histological work was done in the Neurological Laboratory of the Phipps Clinic by Dr. Bartemeier. The work both in Panama and in Baltimore was greatly aided by the interest and encouragement of Dr. Adolf Meyer. (Blass 1976, p. 245)

Richter would study the neurological basis of behavior, and in particular the grasp reflex, for many years. He described his method for studying the grasp reflex in humans as follows:

> The technique of measuring the reflex was similar to that employed in the experiments on the new-born monkeys. The apparatus consisted of two round, parallel brass rods, 1/4 inch (0.6 cm.) in diameter and 5 inches (12.7 cm.) apart, firmly supported 2-1/2 feet (76.3 cm.) above a mattress on a small table. In order to give the infant a firm gripping surface, two short pieces of tight-fitting, thin rubber tubing were placed in the middle of the rods. The infant was held down by the experimenter, just beneath the parallel bars, while an assistant brought the palms of the hands into contact with the bars. As soon as the baby gave any indication of grasping, its body was lowered quickly and it was permitted to hang unsupported. The hanging time recorded with a stopwatch served to measure the strength of the reflex. This method, whereby the infant hangs by both hands rather than by one, has the advantage of eliminating considerable strain, but the hanging time does not seem to be any longer than when the entire weight is supported by one hand. (Richter 1934c, pp. 328–29)

Though Richter noted individual differences and cyclic daily patterns in the grasp reflex, he concluded that it was important for helping newborns cling to their mothers during the neonatal period. He also suggested that the grasp reflex appeared less prominent in humans than in monkeys (Richter 1931a). The method he used with monkeys was different from that used with human newborns, however, so his comparison was misleading. Nonetheless, Richter built on the common evolutionary theme that the grasp reflex was stronger in monkeys than in humans.

Richter chose the sloth for his study of the neural basis of the grasp reflex because the sloth spends most of its time hanging upside down from tree branches (Richter and Bartemeier 1926). Richter's paper described the two- and three-toed sloth (fig. 5.3).

For this study, Richter chose a decerebration method commonly in use at the time (e.g., Bazett and Penfield 1922) to decerebrate a number of sloths. He would later perform the same procedure on other species (e.g., cats, monkeys, beavers).

The decerebrated animal had to be tube-fed to keep it alive, and thermal regulation, like most bodily functions, was compromised. Richter, interested in the organization of posture and of the hanging reflex in particular, noted the compensatory responses that resulted from decerebration-induced motor rigidity. For example, in contrast to decerebration in the cat, which results in extensor rigidity, decerebration in the sloth resulted in flexor rigidity. This was because of the posture of the sloth, in contrast to that of the cat.

Thus Richter predicted, and found evidence, that decerebration leads to exaggerated activity in the antigravity muscles. The rigidity induced by decerebration results from a set of postural reflexes. Richter further noted that tactile stimulation to the head region of the sloth resulted in dissolution of the decerebration-induced flexor rigidity. Richter sought to understand the effects of the decerebration in order to understand the rigidity of limbs in brain-damaged humans. In the case of the sloth, however, decerebration revealed flexor rigidity. In other words, extension rigidity is really antigravity rigidity.

A particular issue with regard to the degree of decerebration-induced rigidity was the role played by the red nucleus (in the brain stem), which had been understood to be essential for posture flexibility. Richter and Bartemeier (1926) noted that their results were consistent with what others had found (e.g., Bazett and Penfield 1922); eleven sloths with transections at the level of the red nucleus showed diminished motor rigidity. The results Richter

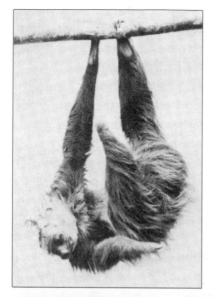
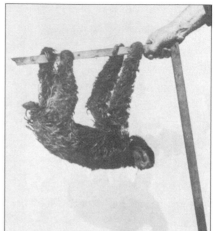

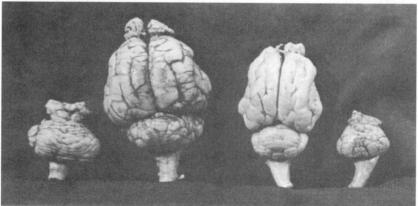

FIG. 5.3. *Top:* Hanging posture of the sloth: *left,* the two-toed sloth; *right,* the three-toed sloth. *Bottom:* The kinds of decerebration performed on each species. *Source:* Richter and Bartemeier 1926

reported also resembled those of Liddell and Sherrington (1924). Richter and Bartemeier (1926) found that the motor rigidity varied with the level of decerebration; if decerebration was above the red nucleus in the brain stem, the rigidity was less pronounced.

Richter was interested in the organization of movement and action. Under the influence of Sherrington, Head, Adrian, Denny-Brown, and other leading neuroscientists of his day, he set out to determine the organization of voluntary and reflex actions, of which the grasp reflex was one. His technique involved using the electromyogram (EMG) to study lesions of the central nervous system.

EMG tests showed that as part of the grasp reflex the flexor muscle of the forearm underwent from five to sixty-five contractions per second, with other wave forms between 180 and 250 per second (Richter 1927b). Richter then inferred that the impulse generators were linked to the wave forms he uncovered in the grasp reflex.

Richter investigated various forms of motor control over behavior, continuing his Jacksonian interest in determining the level of function responsible for the organization of motor control. For example, he looked at the role of motor cortex in decerebrated beavers (Langworthy and Richter 1938). In this electrophysiological study, the researchers recorded responsive neurons in the motor cortex of the beaver and found that stimulation of the frontal cortical areas resulted in movement. This study would again demonstrate one major effect of decerebration, namely, motor rigidity. In this case, the beaver's forelegs were frozen in rigidity.

Richter would continue work on the grasp reflex by observing its physiological and pharmacological basis in a simple study inducing catalepsy by bulbocapnine (Richter and Paterson 1931). It was well known that this agent reduces activity and facilitates catalepsy, causing a great reduction in what Richter and others called "spontaneous movement." He used the drug in macaques, measuring the time an animal could hang with one arm (its other arm and its feet were tied) until it fell to a net. He noted individual differences in response to the injected drug, but the underlying hypothesis was confirmed: the induced catalepsy enhanced the grasp reflex, and the younger the animal, the greater the effect of the drug on the duration of the grasp reflex. The hanging reflex disappeared in adulthood but could be brought on during this drug-induced cataleptic response.

Richter and Paterson looked at the effects on the grasp reflex of injecting various compounds into systemic circulation. In adult macaques, they experimented with over fifteen compounds. The authors found that several of the compounds elicited a grasp reflex in these adults. At high doses, many of these compounds were thought to suppress cerebral activation, especially that related to normal inhibitory input from the motor frontal cortex to the brain stem. In a further study, Richter and Hines showed that frontal lobe lesions in macaques could invoke exaggerated grasplike reflexes in adults (Richter and Hines 1932a).

THE USE OF ELECTRICAL RESISTANCE TO UNDERSTAND NEUROLOGICAL FUNCTION

The very first paper of which Richter was an author reported on a formal technique in which an equilateral triangle was used to predict the electrical patterns of the heart (Carter, Richter, and Greene 1919). The idea of measuring electrical activity was nothing new at this point in physiological inquiry, and Richter would make great use of these electrophysiological techniques for the next fifty years.

Richter next used the EMG to monitor the disruption of voluntary motor control. This avenue of research focused on the amplitude and expression of the EMG wave form in muscles of patients with a diverse range of neurological disorders (e.g., motor horn cell syringomyelia, muscular dystrophy). Richter noted that these diseases often resulted in a reduction or alteration of the wave forms.

In "New Methods of Obtaining Electromyogram and Electrocardiogram from the Intact Body," Richter described his method:

> To obtain records of the action currents from voluntary and reflex contractions of the muscles of the human body, we have devised an electrode that is considerably simpler in construction and manipulation than any of the others commonly employed today. It consists of a sheet of pure zinc about 1 inch square, held in contact with the skin by means of a paste made of kaolin and saturated zinc sulphate solution. This paste alone is sufficient to hold the electrode in place on almost any part of the body; where there is much violent movement of muscles, a large rubber band may also be applied. This electrode has the following advantages: 1) it is non-polarizable; 2) it is quickly and easily prepared; 3) it can be attached over any part of the body, however irregular and inaccessible to other electrodes, and 4) it makes an intimate, moist contact with the skin without producing any irritation or injury even when left in place for several hours. (Richter 1926a, p. 1300)

Richter envisioned the measurement of skin resistance as a basic, broad-based clinical and research tool. He used this method early in his career to measure electrical resistance in skin during sleep (Richter 1926a). At this time, the study of sleep and biological rhythmicity were already a prominent part of Richter's neurological research program. He would attach electrodes to the hand or to other parts of the body, depending on the experiment. In one experiment characterizing the skin resistance of subjects (both humans and macaques) during sleep, he showed that the depth of sleep patterns was correlated with skin resistance in, for instance, the palms of the hands; as the individual began to wake up, the resistance increased.

PSYCHOGALVANIC REFLEXES AND THE AUTONOMIC NERVOUS SYSTEM

Richter's instrumentalist nature again took form in his adaptation of a new tool to measure skin resistance. Meyer had purchased a galvanometer, but the instrument was not being used. Meyer did not like waste. Richter knew that the galvanometer could measure electrical conductivity. He thought surely he could find some use for it, and he did (fig. 5.4).

Interest in measuring skin conductance dated back to the students of Fechner, the father of psychophysics (Richter 1926a). Richter first used the galvanometer to measure skin resistance, which he inferred was an index of the activation of sweat glands in the skin. He then used the device to understand neurological innervations, to detect clinical syndromes, and to determine normal regulatory mechanisms.

Following up on some of the observations Head and his colleagues made of World War I soldiers, Richter sought to reveal the mechanisms of the neural control of sweating. Skin responsiveness and sweating as measures of spinal damage figured significantly in his work over the next two decades, particularly during World War II. The effect of spinal cord transection on the skin galvanic response would lead to an important experimental venture, the rudiments of which were already present in the first part of Richter's neurological investigations (Richter and Shaw 1930).

In one experiment, Richter induced sweating by the simple method of the hot-air bath or by injections of pilocarpine. He also injected atropine into subjects' adrenal glands. He measured sweating from both hands over several months in a patient who had what Richter thought was a unilateral lesion of the sympathetic nervous system (the clinical diagnosis included small pupils and greater-than-normal skin resistance). Measuring what he called the "psychogalvanic reflex" and electrical skin resistance under a variety of conditions, Richter compared the normal side of the body with the damaged side. Atropine produced no effect on the damaged side, but the psychogalvanic reflex was eliminated or altered on the side with damage. Richter took this as proof of the role of the sympathetic nervous system in this response (Richter 1927c).

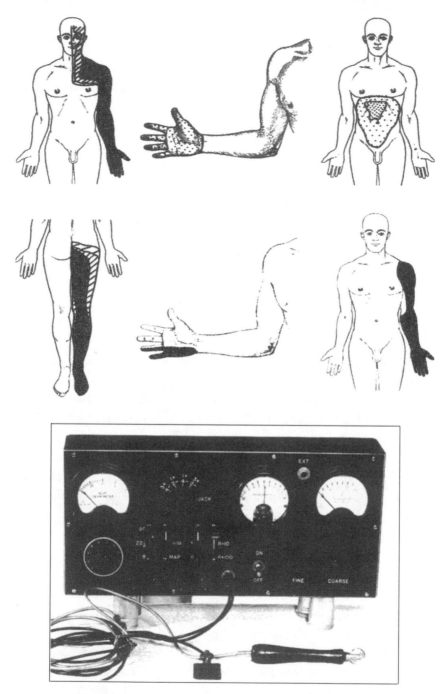

FIG. 5.4. *Top*: Skin conductance as a measure of nerve injury. *Bottom*: A dermometer.
Source: Richter 1947; Riley and Richter 1975

Richter and his neurological colleagues almost always provided a fairly detailed depiction of the patients in their experiments. Each pathological group usually consisted of one or two subjects. The researchers' methods resembled a clinical case study more than a true experimental design, and the results were typically presented as case vignettes with an experimental bent.

In further studies, Richter continued to look at the relationship between neuromuscular damage and various reflexes. This research emphasized the relationship between the brain and peripheral systemic regulation. Richter and Ford used the EMG to determine wave forms and their link to muscular activity. They found a reduction in primary wave forms among patients with hypothesized lesions of the motor horn, syringomyelia, muscular atrophy, and poliomyelitis, although the amplitude was still large despite the atrophied musculature (Richter and Ford 1928).

In an experiment with macaques and cats, Richter cut various nerves to determine the effect on skin resistance. For example, he cut the somatic nerves, leaving intact what he thought was the sympathetic system in three monkeys and five cats. This resulted in changes in skin resistance. In another experiment, Richter surgically removed the abdominal sympathetic nervous system, leaving the somatic nerves intact (Richter 1929b). Because he provided no histologic data, it is difficult to determine the accuracy of his procedures. He did report that he performed a histological examination, however. The effect of the sympathectomy was to initiate an increase in conductivity in the porous regions of the skin, which then gradually decreased over time. Richter articulated the view that the sympathetic ganglia regulated skin conductivity and that reciprocal innervations of sympathetic and parasympathetic systems regulated systemic physiological end-organ systems.

Richter went on to examine the relationship between sleep and electrical skin resistance, again looking at the hand. He found that average skin resistance was higher in patients with muscular pathology than in normal control subjects and that there was wider variation in resistance in patients with damaged spinal cords. Comparing these results with those from several other clinically pathological states, such as schizophrenic stupor, he found his results to be most similar to those in narcoleptic patients. He speculated that the disruption of sleep patterns in narcolepsy might reflect an "encephalitic process" (Richter 1929c).

The sympathetic nervous system and the recovery response would be a constant neurological interest of Richter's (Tower and Richter 1932a, 1932b).

Richter and his colleagues examined patient populations with sympathetic damage at the Johns Hopkins Hospital (Richter and Levine 1937). They performed cervical sympathectomies at different levels among four patient populations (those with migraine, neuralgia, Hirschsprung disease, and Raynaud disease). In each case, after the sympathectomy, skin resistance was increased.

CLINICAL ASSESSMENT OF WAR WOUNDS
IN WORLD WAR II SOLDIERS

During World War II, Richter found himself with a useful technique for monitoring neurological damage in soldiers. As noted earlier, he had inherited the galvanometer from Meyer, and now he developed and expanded its use, devising a smaller version of this tool that would facilitate his collaboration with several colleagues in the field of neurology (e.g., Tower, Levine, and Katz) and allow him to embark on new neurological studies.

Richter's laboratory state of mind led him to take advantage of an opportunity to use his new instrument with World War II soldiers. Richter, the scavenger-scientist, always made the most of whatever was available, inventing simple tools and using simple measuring techniques to great effect. He epitomized the tenacity of the scientist by continuing to apply and extend his methods to determine their full usefulness.

Richter noted early on that some forms of bodily damage altered skin conductance, and he continued to develop methods to determine the relationship between sensory processing and sympathetic damage (Richter 1926a). One common theme in this research was the link between high resistance in electrical conductivity and diminished sweat (Richter and Woodruff 1941).

Having developed a small, portable galvanometer they called a "dermometer," Richter and his colleagues measured skin resistance (Whelan and Richter 1943; Richter 1946b) and extended the dermometer's use to determine peripheral bodily damage (Richter and Whelan 1949). Identifying areas in the hand and foot with differences in electrical skin resistance, Richter, Woodruff, and Eaton (1943) further explored the link between skin resistance and sweating.

In the *Journal of the American Medical Association* at the height of World War II, Richter and Katz, in their most publicized statement, described their line of research as having three primary goals: (1) to determine anatomically the areas innervated by peripheral nerves, (2) to discern damaged areas, and (3) to note neural regeneration and recovery. In one experiment, they found increased electrical skin resistance after injections of procaine were used to block the nerve in question. They asserted: "The simplicity, accuracy and speed of the method make it useful for the exact examination of all types of peripheral nerve lesions" (Richter and Katz 1943, p. 651).

Further studies by Richter and his colleagues in the immediate postwar period further helped to ascertain the mechanisms of sweating and skin resistance. The researchers labored under the influence of Langley and Sherrington in determining which sympathetic fibers were important for the response. Richter collaborated on studies in monkeys (Bruesch and Richter 1946) and humans (Richter and Otenasek 1946), looking at different regions of the body under various experimental conditions after different kinds of sympathectomies. The results, on the whole, tended to reflect greater electrical skin resistance in patients with denervated regions.

Richter's work in this area was supported by colleagues, mostly clinical medical doctors (e.g., Maurice Levine). They hoped he could parlay the use of the galvanic instrument into a broadly useful clinical instrument, one that could be supported by the military in the war effort (Bump 1996).

So it was that during the war Richter and his colleagues continued to look at a number of clinical populations with the portable dermometer. He continued to note great variations in skin resistance in the populations he studied (Richter and Otenasek 1946). Richter and his students and colleagues were on the offensive to persuade the military of the usefulness of his technique to detect peripheral pathology (Bump 1996). Richter would, in fact, effectively promote his instruments and his methodology in some cases; for example, Surling at Walter Reed Army Medical Center was persuaded of the clinical utility of the tool. Although Richter secured military contracts for his research, military physicians were divided in their opinions of the method. With variation in results and diminished prospects for its utility as a general tool, use of the dermometer began to wane (Bump 1996).

Nonetheless, Richter and his colleagues continued to publish papers on the use of electrical skin resistance as a measure of peripheral neurological damage. Into the 1960s, he would think of the skin resistance method as a way to detect pathology (see Fries and Richter 1964).

TENACITY

Richter always looked for ways to extend the use of a method or tool to other applications and areas of study. In the early 1930s he extended his study of electrical skin resistance to the study of mental illness. Looking at electrical resistance of the skin "in catatonic and depressive stupors and similar conditions . . . to determine whether it is possible to separate these conditions on the basis of skin resistance," Richter inquired into "experimental catatonia" (Meyer files, Chesney Archives). He became interested in "measuring the postural changes characteristic of catatonia," using this measure to understand "the grasping reflex," and using high and low electrical resistance to discern catatonia's neurological basis in sympathetic and peripheral damage (Richter 1946b; Richter, Woodruff, and Eaton 1943).

Some fifty years after his first publication on the use of the electrode to measure skin resistance, and with long periods in which this experimental issue was not at the forefront of his laboratory or clinical concerns, Richter returned to the topic. Never one to leave something behind, he summarized in a paper what he took to be the underlying principles of his technique:

> The neurological and physiological principles underlying use of this method were worked out 1924–1934 on cats, monkeys, and human subjects: 1. Passage of a direct electrical current through the body is localized practically entirely in the skin. 2. Electrical skin resistance reflects activity of the sweat glands, but not of actual amounts of sweat. 3. Heat lowers the electrical resistance of the skin; cold increases it. 4. Sectioning of peripheral nerves increases skin resis-tance; irritation of peripheral nerves decreases it. 5. Sympathectomy increases skin resistance; hyperactivity of sympathetic nerves decreases it. 6. Depression increases; emotional excitement increases it. (Riley and Richter 1975, pp. 59–60)

In the 1970s, Richter was still applying this method, in collaboration with clinicians, to determine whether skin electrical resistance was associated with pain in the neck and upper extremities (Richter 1972; Riley and Richter 1975).

CONCLUSION

Richter was an adventurous spirit; he grew up in the outdoors. It was not surprising that early in his career he would make a sojourn to Central America. Following the naturalists of the nineteenth and early twentieth centuries, he embarked on a brief excursion to study animals near their natural habitat. He still investigated with a laboratory state of mind; he just did it closer to, and sometimes in, the animals' natural environment.

The influence of Theodore Roosevelt pervaded the Panama Canal, which he was responsible for having built. F. M. Chapman, a leading figure from the American Museum of Natural History who spent time on Barro Colorado

Island, commented, "Always in the background stands the figure of Theodore Roosevelt, who whether on the Zone or in the White House, was the inspiring, understanding leader" (Chapman 1938, p. 4). Roosevelt was a naturalist, founder of the Museum of Natural History, and a conservationist. He revered nature and science and brought great projects to fruition. Perhaps Richter embraced the idea of President Roosevelt, a rugged individual with an appreciation of natural resources, a can-do attitude, a lot of muscle, and little fear.

Richter inherited his interest in the grasp reflex from Watson and studied it primarily to understand the neurology and the pharmacology that made it possible. Richter remained rooted in a neurological tradition in which evolution permeated the conception of the brain. The hierarchical conception of the nervous system was, and still is, a common intellectual framework for understanding the brain. Richter inherited this perspective and used it creatively in his own investigations. This research also demonstrated his long-term focus on core issues and the development and pragmatic use of research tools.

With increasing age and prestige, Richter never seemed to discard the old tools but continued to expand their application. Though not atheoretical, Richter engaged first and foremost with experiments, inventions, and the practical meanings of science. Richter retained pervasive interests in the neurological techniques and data he generated and in the methods he used. As in the case of the clinical dermometer, he constantly returned to and revised his methods.

CHAPTER 6

An Artisan in the Laboratory

There are traditions of inquiry that radically separate thought from the activities of the artisan and theory from the mundane work of the laboratory. In these traditions, the knower is on one side and the artificer on the other. This view has been criticized by many (e.g., Dewey 1934/1958; Hollinger 1994), and I believe it is a misleading way of understanding much of science. A scientist more at home at the level of invention of instruments may be simultaneously embedded in theory and invested in experiment (Galison 1988).

Curt Richter, though he probably never articulated it, understood the fallacy of this dichotomous view of inquiry. Richter was always involved with the creation of knowledge and the discovery of new facts.

A HANDS-ON APPROACH

Richter found ingenious ways to study phenomena. A quote displayed in Richter's laboratory was attributed to François Magendie, the father of experimental physiology and Bernard's teacher: "Everyone compares himself to something more or less majestic in his own sphere, to Archimedes, Michelangelo, Galileo, Descartes, and so on. Louis XIV compared himself to the sun. I am much more humble. I compare myself to a scavenger; with my book in my hand and my pack on my back, I go about the domain of science, picking up what I can find" (Rozin 1976a, p. xviii).

Richter was a scientific scavenger-entrepreneur. The experiment dominated his conception of what it meant to be a psychobiologist. Richter's world was rich in scientific breadth and invention; it was the world of the artisan scientist, the maker of tools. His sensibility can be traced to those of modern experimenters like Robert Boyle, who understood experimentation as vitally important to understanding science and to the trust that is afforded the things we claim to know (Shapin and Schaffer 1985). Most scientists live in a world in which instruments are shared. As Galison (1987) made clear, the shared instruments link various experiments. Richter loved the invention of new tools and new instruments.

Science does not take place in a vacuum; it requires a culture of inquiry, artifacts, and labor. Peirce wrote elegantly about the community of inquirers, about the way a proposition's meaning is defined by the broad array of experimental and conceptual tests it undergoes, and about investigators having as a normative goal the culmination of their opinions in truth (Peirce 1877, 1878, 1898/1992).

Richter considered existing ideas in physiology and psychobiology and devised ways to study them in the laboratory. Richter did not, for example, invent the concept of wisdom of the body popularized by Cannon; rather, Richter made it a laboratory artifact, something studied or realized in the laboratory. Neither did he invent the idea of biological clocks or of domestication of internal physiology and behavior, but he made them suitable objects for laboratory study.

THE STRUCTURE OF THE LABORATORY

The structure of the laboratory, its organization, its products, and its forces of production make up a subfield of study for the historian of science (see Latour and Woolgar 1979/1986). The laboratory setting, of course, can not be contained within an unequivocal definition. There is no platonic definition of a laboratory, just the common depiction of an investigator instantiating and studying, controlling and understanding an object of study. Richter might have agreed with this description of a laboratory setting: "Laboratories allow natural processes to be 'brought home'" (Cetina 1999, p. 29). Of course, some phenomena brought into the laboratory may become artifacts of the laboratory; by definition, experimental science does not allow for the study of unadulterated nature (see Kohler 2002). For all the analysis that, for example, Latour and Woolgar (1979/1986) provide in their book *Laboratory Life,* they never seem close to capturing a sense of the laboratory in which playfulness, or for that matter, the artisan sensibility (Lynch 1985), is expressed. Richter surely was productive, focused, and driven, but he enjoyed his collaborators, the creation of useful tools for measurement, and the esthetic creations of laboratory life.

NOT ALONE, BUT A LONER

Richter was a loner and eschewed the usual role of an academic, avoiding, for example, academic meetings when at all possible. He never worked in a typical university setting. He had few graduate and undergraduate students, but this does not mean that he worked alone. He maintained long-term relationships with his research staff and with some of his colleagues (e.g., Eliot Stellar).

A laboratory community can have a familial feeling, though certainly this is not always the case. Like families, laboratories differ in the degree to which they are benign or nurturing for their individual members. Richter appears to have engendered a congenial ambiance in which individuals could participate in the culture of science and in a laboratory life devoted to the production of scientific facts, the testing of ideas, and the exploring of biological matters that had an impact on human health.

Of course, Richter made the most of his staff's allegiance and loyalty in order to produce well-conducted research. Research takes place in a social context, with individuals who have different interests and levels of commitment. But always Richter was the man in charge, the leader of his laboratory.

STUDENTS AND COLLABORATORS

Richter had very few Ph.D. students, but he did have a cadre of medical students who worked on projects with him in his laboratory. He also had a few colleagues who began their careers working with him and remained with him for long periods.

Several of the medical students who worked in Richter's laboratory were Henry Strong Denison scholars at Hopkins. Many of the papers Richter wrote were coauthored with these medical students. Indeed, medical students, together with key technicians, were staples of his laboratory (Keiner 1996).

Particularly important colleagues included Sally Dieke, who earned a Ph.D. in chemistry, and Katherine Rice, who received her M.D. from Hopkins. Rice worked with Richter principally on the specific hungers and was an active member of his laboratory intermittently from 1941 to 1957, while she worked as a practicing psychiatrist.

During the most productive periods in Richter's laboratory (from the end of the 1930s through the 1940s), Bruno Barelare and John Eckert, who each earned an M.D. and worked on the specific hungers, stood out as particularly productive coauthors. Several individuals who worked in the Psychobiology Laboratory as research associates had Ph.D.s (e.g., Wang, Kinder, Dieke, and M. Hines). Other noteworthy colleagues were E. Holt, M.D. (a professor of pediatrics), and O. Langworthy, M.D. (a professor of neurology).

It is unclear from Richter's work which ideas were his and which belonged to his colleagues and students. It is clear that they helped him and that he had long-term relationships with several key laboratory colleagues. In some instances they lent a technical hand; in others, they tested an idea in which Richter was particularly interested.

In his autobiography (Richter 1985), Richter included the following acknowledgments: "Over the past sixty years, many medical students and members of the hospital and medical school staffs collaborated in these researches: Katherine Rice, Sally Dieke, Carl Hartman, Bruno Barelare, John Eckert, Douglas Hawkes, E. Schmidt, Emmett Holt, and David Mosier" (Richter 1985).

Several key colleagues at the beginning of his career were essential to his initial successes, and a long list of influential individuals held Richter in high regard. Those who worked with him seemed quite devoted to him.

David Mosier worked with Richter on the contrast between wild and domestic rats (on end-organ systems) over several summers in the late 1940s and early 1950s. Mosier worked with Richter at Hopkins while he was a medical student and then again when he returned as a resident in endocrinology (1955–57). Mosier described Richter in this way: "He seemed to go on in that third-floor laboratory as if it was given to him by God. He exuded so much confidence. But then again, perhaps he was given the laboratory by God" (D. Mosier, pers. comm., February 2003).

Mosier described Richter as unpretentious and helpful to the medical students who worked in his laboratory, offering them gentle criticism and encouragement. Mosier also remarked that toward the end of his life, the tired Richter perked up when he learned of Mosier's involvement with a large primate facility, responding, "My God, David, that is fantastic." Richter was always excited by the prospect of research, even at the end, and he extended that enthusiasm to others.

LABORATORY STAFF

Richter also formed long-lasting relationships with the technical workers in his laboratory. Technical support was vital for Richter's investigations, as it is for many investigators (see Shapin 1989). Many of his technical helpers worked with him for years, and when I interviewed several of them, including Ardis O'Connor and Barbara Carberry Cross, they expressed their devotion to Richter and talked about how they kept the laboratory going and felt that they were part of a great enterprise. Richter would never have been as productive as he was without the laboratory staff he cultivated over a long period. Individuals like O'Connor, Cross, and Agnes Molloy kept the laboratory alive and working, and many saw their careers as defined by being part of the Richter laboratory.

Richter trained the members of his laboratory staff to serve in a variety of functions. For example, Peg Brunner and Ardis O'Connor helped with activity charts. Several technicians, including Ardis O'Connor and M. Eckman, developed a level of competence that allowed them to participate in surgical procedures. These people had such a sense of commitment to Richter that, even in his last years, those who had gone on to other positions still helped and remained loyal to him (A. O'Connor and B. Carberry Cross, pers. comm., June 2003).

Ardis O'Connor worked with Richter for more than thirty years, from 1944 to 1978, and she and Richter performed countless surgical operations together (A. O'Connor, pers. comm., June 2003). Richter said of O'Connor: "For nearly thirty-three years, Mrs. O'Connor had complete responsibility for the maintenance of standard conditions in all of my experiments and also was in charge of my colony of Norway rats" (Richter 1985, p. 386). Like many successful scientists, Richter engendered commitment and devotion from a variety of individuals involved in the scientific enterprise.

RICHTER'S LABORATORY IN CONTEXT

The importance of inventing methods, though now obvious, once needed to be stated by scientists such as Bernard and Pavlov, who celebrated the laboratory methods that moved the science of physiology beyond simple observation (Holmes 1974; Todes 2002). Richter was very much in this tradition but lacked the public demeanor Bernard and Pavlov had. He was happy to be sequestered in the laboratory, to enjoy the sweet success of an accomplished scientist, and to relish the cultural life of the Baltimore elite class.

Richter's laboratory was less structured than Pavlov's, which was characterized by Daniel Todes, a scientific historian, as a behavioral or physiological factory. In a fairly positive and detailed depiction of the workings of Pavlov's laboratory, Todes documented the production of scientific facts that emerged from the structure of that laboratory.

Pavlov is well known in the scientific community and was a Nobel laureate. Richter, in contrast, was not as distinguished an intellectual figure as was Pavlov, Cannon, or even Karl Lashley. He was much less famous and had far fewer students and colleagues working in his laboratory. He was, however, very much appreciated by core individuals, was seen as a serious investigator, and had gathered the major trimmings of scientific success.

And Richter was playful. His mode of inquiry reflected that fact. Discovery and invention and the free rein of exploration predominated. He could be jovial and stubborn at the same time. Whereas Pavlov was on a crusade through his science, Richter was a playful laboratory artisan. Although he was the leader of his laboratory, by all accounts his manner had a light touch. The little boy who tinkered on the floor of his mother's factory never really departed. Pavlov would not have handed out greeting cards of rats ingesting sucrose (see fig. 3.5). Consider the title of Richter's autobiographical reminiscences: "It's a Long Way to Tipperary, the Land of My Genes" (Richter 1985). Would Pavlov ever have used such a title? Surely not! Despite his playfulness in the laboratory, however, Richter was always serious and disciplined about his work.

Richter remained an engineer/experimentalist to the core. Entering his laboratory, one experienced the vitality and creativity that permeated the space. The master craftsman was revealed through the elegance of his laboratory, his adroit use of space, and the placement of his charts and surgical tools. Richter's artisan sensibilities were apparent.

AN UNFINISHED PROJECT: THE RICHTER-MALONE BOOK

Just as Richter often depended on others to keep his laboratory going and lend him their hands and minds, he teamed up with a particular laboratory artisan to work out his surgical depictions. Richter's collaboration with Paul Malone was an important one. Malone was a medical illustrator who had studied with Max Brödel, assisting the great illustrator on drawings of the inner ear (Brödel 1946; Crosby and Cody 1991), and he eventually became the director of medical illustration at the Lahey Clinic Foundation in Boston.

Max Brödel worked with many people at Hopkins, including William Stewart Halsted and Harvey Cushing, both noted surgeons who greatly influenced Richter (the work of Halsted on surgical parathyroidectomy is one example; see Crowe 1957). An artist who had trained in Leipzig with the physiologist Carl Ludwig, Brödel was a legendary figure at Hopkins. He arrived at Hopkins from Germany in 1894, and by 1911 he had created the Department of Art as

Applied to Medicine (Schultheiss and Jonas 1999), where he would serve as director for nearly thirty years (Cullen 1945). Brödel stated his position clearly: "A medical picture, correctly planned and accurately and artistically executed, is an integral part of the medical literature" (Brödel 1941, p. 668). In fact, anatomical art had been established centuries earlier as an integral part of the medical sciences. The notebooks of Leonardo da Vinci are full of drawings of conceptual possibilities (flying machines), realistic medical dissections, and glorious art tied to a philosophy of exploration and experimentation (da Vinci 1980). Da Vinci's emphasis was on art, on simulation, on the building of things. In his day, there was no separation between art and practicality; the everyday utility an artisan created through perspective and ingenuity was appreciated (Dewey 1934/1958). Art was central to medical depiction.

When Richter and Malone set out to publish a book on rat surgery, W. B. Saunders Publishing Company expressed interest. In 1972, Malone wrote to Richter that "[Saunders] agree we write a book if you can finish it up in 6 months" (Richter files, Chesney Archives, June 23, 1972). Malone noted in the same letter that "you and I both know that circumstances are such that we cannot continue to add drawings." Some five years later, Malone wrote to a colleague that "we hope to publish the rat surgery eventually." Richter noted that "surgery has always given me particular pleasure. I still do all the operating on my animals and all autopsies. Ordinarily I spend almost half my time operating—am still able to perform almost every operation on a rat that can be done on dogs or man, with the exception of those on blood vessels. I am hoping shortly to publish (with P. D. Malone, a medical artist) a full description of all of these operations in a book on 'Experimental Surgery of the Rat'" (Richter files, Chesney Archives).

The next several figures are examples of Richter's and Malone's surgical/anatomical drawings. Richter and his colleagues conducted a number of their behavioral studies with an emphasis on the importance of the oral cavity (fig. 6.1) and the gustatory nerves, including several of the cranial nerves (fig. 6.2). Figures 6.3 and 6.4 depict two of Richter's experimental techniques: the removal of the pituitary gland and a retinal implant in a rat, respectively.

Richter described his work with Malone as follows:

This great collection of drawings of surgical operations and maneuvers on the Norway rat resulted from many happy years of collaboration with Mr. P. D. Malone, now one of the leading medical illustrators in this country. There never has been anything to equal these drawings—lovely to look at even without any knowledge

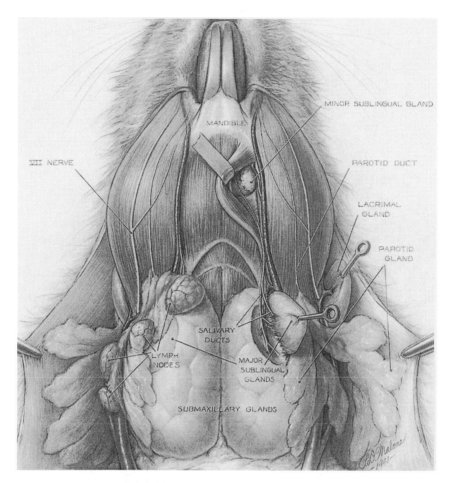

FIG. 6.1. Glands associated with the oral cavity. *Source:* Alan Mason Chesney Medical Archives, Johns Hopkins Medical Institutions

or main interest. My contribution was minor. I merely designed the operations needed for the various experiments and did the operations. In preparation for making the drawings, Mr. Malone and I worked very closely together, constantly checking and re-checking each other's versions until finally we felt satisfied that the drawings gave an accurate and complete account of each operation.

Mr. Malone started his career with Max Brödel, the first medical illustrator in this country, and became an expert in the use of the Brödel technique. Brödel took a keen and active interest in the drawings that Mr. Malone made for my experiments and offered many helpful criticisms and suggestions. Mr. Malone's drawings gave Brödel much pleasure and satisfaction. (Richter files, Chesney Archives)

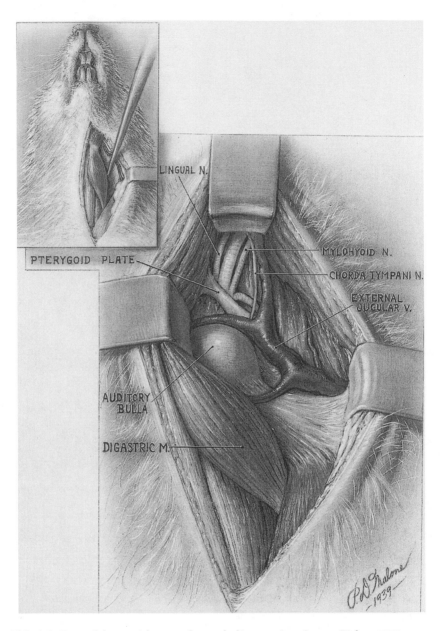

FIG. 6.2. Parts of the cranial nerves that underlie gustation. *Source:* Richter 1956

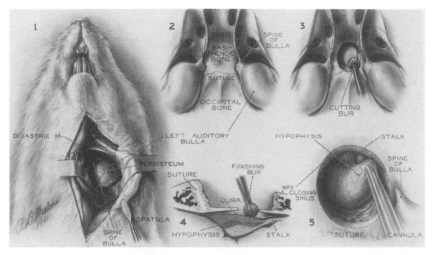

FIG. 6.3. Steps in removing the pituitary gland of a rat. *Source:* Alan Mason Chesney Medical Archives, Johns Hopkins Medical Institutions

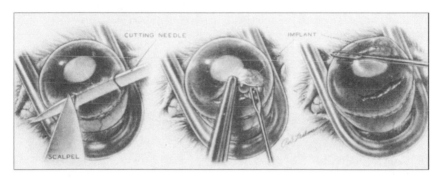

FIG. 6.4. The surgical techniques used to implant tissue in the anterior chamber of the eye. *Source:* Richter 1956

Richter and Malone envisioned many possible chapters for their book. Table 6.1 lists suggested illustrations (Richter files, Chesney Archives). Unfortunately, the work was never published, for unknown reasons, perhaps a waning interest on the part of the publisher. The illustrations remain in the Richter files at the Chesney Archives, perhaps to be rediscovered and used one day by others.

Richter's heart as a scientist, his pride as the artisan scientist, and his long-term relationships are evident in his work on the illustrations. He loved this aspect of the science; he enjoyed building, describing, and diagramming a

TABLE 6.1. Partial List of Illustrations in Richter and Malone's
Unpublished Book Proposal

Surgical Anatomy of the Rat: Illustrations of Operations or Dissections

1. Exposure of all the Endocrine Glands (Photographs, Drawings)
2. Removal of Kidney Capsules, Adrenals and Accessory Adrenal Nodules
3. Accessory Adrenal Nodule
4. Sagittal Section of the Brain Showing Location of Stab Wound Near Hypothalamus
5. Removal of the Pituitary
6. Method of Holding Mouth Open for Insertion of Tracheal Cannula
7. Bands in Rat's Throat in Preparation for Insertion of Cannula
8. Blood Vessel Supply to All Lobes of Pancreas
9. Four Steps Involved in the Total Removal of the Pancreas
10. Distention of Cecum in Pancreatectomized Rat
11. Condition of Cornea in Pancreatectomized Diabetic Rat
12. Removal of the Parathyroid Glands
13. Three Steps Involved in Implanting Tissue in the Anterior Chamber of the Eye
14. Three of the First Steps Involved in the Panhysterectomy
15. Last Three Steps of the Panhysterectomy
16. Lobes of Liver, Stomach, Duodenum, Pancreas, Colon
17. Hepatectomy
18. Greatly Distended Lymph Vessels following Tube Feeding with Olive Oil
19. Distention of Lymphatic Ducts following Injection of Animal with Milk
20. Thoratic-Lymphatic Ducts
21. Peyer's Patch on Intestine of Domestic Norway Rats
22. Removal of the Lung
23. Pneumenectomy
24. Dissection of the Taste Nerves
25. Further Dissection of Taste Nerves
26. Cross-Sections of Taste Bud and Papillae and Tongue Surface
27. Circumvalate Papillae
28. Sectioning of Optic Nerve
29. Various Neck Glands
30. Salivary Glands
31. Skull and Brain Stem Stub
32. Operating Stand
33. Removal of Superior Cervical Ganglion
34. Tube Feeding
35. Brain of Rats, Chipmunk, etc.
36. Cancer Eating
37. Pituitary Tumor
38. Bile Duct
39. Holding Rat for Abdominal Injection
40. Nest Building
41. Activity and Brain Operations
42. Parathyroidectomy and Brain Operations
43. Gastrectomy
44. Ovarian Transplant
45. Seminal Vesicles and Prostate
46. Thymus

useful experimental product, in this case anatomical and surgical drawings. Epistemological advances, for Richter, often were based on the practical, artisan side of science.

CONCLUSION

Richter approached his laboratory life with an artisan sensibility, evident in the instruments he used, in the simplicity of his experimentation, and, of course, in his results. Richter's collaboration with Malone was indicative of the fact that he loved simple inventions, whether an elegant anatomical drawing or an experimental manipulation that translated into interesting data. He was a laboratory scientist who took pleasure in the esthetic aspects of everyday activities. Although Richter and Malone do not equal Leonardo da Vinci, Richter's relationship with Malone resulted in a mutually beneficial and productive partnership. The object to be depicted, in the hands of these two craftsmen, was enhanced by their mutual effort. Richter knew what he wanted, and Malone knew how to produce it.

Richter described his relationship to Malone as follows: "For his years in my laboratory we had a wonderful working relationship. I showed him how I did an operation; he made a drawing; then I checked the drawing; and then we continued this exchange until we felt certain that the drawings gave an accurate picture of all the details. In many instances Mr. Malone not only made the drawings, but gave helpful suggestions for improving the operation" (Richter files, Chesney Archives, February 21, 1978).

A laboratory state of mind is one in which measurement predominates. In the Roe interviews, for example, when asked about his thinking process, Richter tellingly said, "I would say that I think really very little in terms of words. I think largely in terms of moving my hands. I find that I am always about 10 steps behind in my verbalizations." A little later he is quoted as saying, "I have a passion, I suppose, for measuring things" (Roe interview notes, American Philosophical Society Archives, 1952).

Anne Roe commented on her interview with Richter, "At this point we went through his labs and had a look at the rats, wild and domestic, and all of the fancy equipment which he has. It's a staggering place as far as set-up goes— small, tightly organized" (Roe interviews, American Philosophical Society Archives, 1962). His laboratory was a thing of beauty—a place lived fully.

One forgets at times that esthetic sensibility did not evolve first for those most cherished artifacts of our culture such as great paintings; instead, it was trapped in the trenches of the commonplace, equated with mundane objects like household pottery, for example. In his book *Art as Experience,* Dewey went to great lengths to outline the "fulfillment of an organism in its struggles and achievements" as containing "the promise of that delightful perception which is aesthetic experience" (Dewey 1934/1958, p. 18). Esthetics, in this account, one that I embrace, is tied to our human ability to resolve problems, depict events, invent, and discover. There is no separation between functionality and esthetics in the laboratory, where an anatomical depiction of surgery, a guide for transplants, and a simple tool can all be esthetically pleasing. Esthetics is part of the human experience of invention and discovery.

Richter was lucky to have worked mostly in an age before "big science" would come to undermine what he romanticized as "free science," but in the 1950s the era of big grant writing was at hand. Now, Richter lamented, to get a grant one had to know in advance what one was going to find out (1953f). Exploration and play, he feared, would be lost, and scientific creativity would be compromised.

Richter prided himself on his surgical abilities. He remarked to a number of people who knew him (e.g., Epstein, Stellar, and Wolf) about his surgical prowess. Eliot Vallenstein, a psychobiologist at the University of Michigan, recalled a time when Richter was applying for a grant. He pleaded with the review committee not to let his age (he was in his late seventies) affect their judgment; he needed the money for his assistant who had been with him for many years. Moreover, he said, "my eyes are clear, my hands are steady, and I have performed 784 operations this year" (E. Vallenstein, pers. comm., July 2002).

Although he was never part of mainstream psychology, within the field of psychology Richter is typically associated with the concept of drive. One noted historian of psychology in the United States described Richter as "a persistent and ingenious experimenter" (Hilgard 1987). Individuals such as Neal Miller, who was himself part of mainstream psychology, seem to have been quite impressed with Richter. But Richter rarely interacted with psychologists.

Conclusion

Curt Richter envisioned himself and his work as part of the scientific enlight-enment. In Richter's words, "We are participants in a great revolutionary movement." The contents of science matter for the human condition; science has practical consequences. Again in Richter's words, "We as scientists are beginning to hold the responsibility for the future in our own hands" (Richter 1953f, p. 91). Although Richter was not a public intellectual, certainly not in the sense of Meyer or Watson or Cannon, he did seem to understand his work in the context of the larger social milieu.

Richter assumed a broad view of biological adaptation. For him, the con-cept of instinct was a behavioral category for animals' orientation to the world in which problem solving takes place. He thought, as he would always say, with his hands, with instruments of measurement. Richter exemplified a research program richly conceived within regulatory physiology and biologi-cal adaptation.

An important conference that Richter attended toward the end of the 1950s provides a context for Richter's insistence on staying focused on the concrete, practical application of scientific inquiry while remaining apart from the intellectual and theoretical debates of his day.

AN INTERNATIONAL CONFERENCE ON INSTINCTIVE BEHAVIOR

A conference on the concept of instinct and metabolism was organized by French scientists and held in France a little more than a decade after World War II. This international conference brought together an interesting group of European and American investigators. Participants included Konrad Lorenz,

Daniel Lehrman, K. Von Frisch, T. C. Schneirla, and Desmond Morris, among others. This lively group submitted papers that resulted in the publication in French of *L'instinct dans le comportement des animaux et de l'homme.*

As I have indicated, instinct is a fundamental concept in psychobiology. It was also an important concept for Richter; one of his review articles, "Salt Appetite of Mammals: Its Dependence on Instinct and Metabolism," featured instinct as a central factor in salt appetite (Richter 1956d). The concept of instinct, in fact, pervades all of Richter's work.

At the conference, the stage was set for a confrontation between Lorenz and a young, vociferous critic of his work, Daniel Lehrman. Lehrman had earlier published "A Critique of Konrad Lorenz's Theory of Instinctive Behavior," in which he argued that Lorenz's notion of instinctive behavior, as innate releasing patterns of behavioral expression, was far too narrow. Moreover, Lehrman argued that innate constraints are not the same across species, and that the concept of instinct used to explain behavior was easily abused. Rather, there were variations in the degree to which behavior and responses to specific stimuli were fixed among different species. How much they varied, as well as how much they were a characteristic of a given species and its evolutionary ascent, had not been answered by ethology. Lehrman argued for greater plasticity at the level of the brain and behavior, which is certainly a feature of human beings (Lehrman 1953).

Lorenz, in his paper at the conference, presented "the objectivist theory of instinct" and defended his position against Lehrman, particularly his hydraulic model of the build-up of drive and its release to specific stimuli. Lehrman challenged Lorenz's ideas on specific points, particularly on issues of ontogeny (Lorenz 1956). Others also spoke out. There is no record of how Richter may have weighed in on this discussion.

Other papers presented at the conference were less theoretical. Although many of the speakers at the conference asked questions during the discussion, there is no record of comments from Richter. Finally, after a talk by Desmond Morris on "the function and causation of courtship ceremonies," Richter asked a question: "Is a surgical attack on a behavior problem possible in the fish, as it is in mammals, for instance, the rat? It would be of considerable importance to know how removal of the various endocrine glands would alter the behavior of your fish; or how isolated brain lesions would alter them. Do fish have a sufficiently high resistance to infections to permit surgical interferences to be made without endangering their lives?" (Grasse, p. 285).

Other papers followed, some of which were very empirical discussions of the physiological and behavioral regulation of different forms of adaptation. Many of these papers were in French or German. Recall that Richter understood German and could also speak it. A paper by Schneirla, "Interrelationships of the 'Innate' and the 'Acquired' in Instinctive Behavior," again emphasized ontogeny, as the American naturalists tended to study each species on its own ecological terms. Schneirla stated in his conclusion that he wanted to "retire" the concept of instinct from the scientific lexicon (Schneirla 1956). This conference is one of the few instances in which there was direct interaction between the American naturalists from the Museum of Natural History (Schneirla, Lehrman), and Lorenz, a German soldier from the war, distinguished naturalist, and eventual Nobel Prize winner and one of the grand promoters of the concept of instinct. This was not just about science; it was personal.

Interestingly, in Lehrman's essay "On the Organization of Maternal Behavior and the Problem of Instinct," he included a good deal of discussion on the hormonal regulation of maternal behavior (Lehrman 1956). In this paper Lehrman emphasized the interaction between hormonal regulation of behavior and experience and how experience modified behavior (*experience* here referred to a concept larger than that of associative learning).

This paper indicated that Lehrman was well acquainted with some of Richter's work; he cited both Richter and Kinder on the behavioral regulation of temperature through nest building. Lehrman also cited the work of Wada and Richter and that of Richter on stomach contractions and the regulation of activity and food intake. Lehrman's main focus, however, was Lorenz. Although one wonders what Richter thought of it all, there is no record of this. Perhaps he was right to stay out of the ideological debate. At the conference, Richter would stick to discussing one of his favorite topics: the appetite for salt.

Richter, appearing unmoved by the theoretical shouts at this conference, gave one of his best presentations on the innate mechanisms that underlie salt ingestion. He showed that salt appetite was dependent on two factors: instinct and metabolism. By *instinct* he meant innate behavioral expression, and by *metabolism* he meant the physiological mechanisms that generate behavior and preserve sodium balance.

The issue of innateness had long been settled for Richter. Although clearly he knew of the debates about the role of innate and learned behaviors and their interactions in ingestive behavior, as well as the ideological debates that plagued the use of the concept of instinct, he no doubt was happy not to engage. Perhaps, although he never really asserted this, he would happily dissolve the distinction that some held between instinct and intelligence, the former blind and automatic and the latter adaptive and subject to trial and error (see Boakes 1984).

The argument Richter put forth was that "studies on salt appetite which we have carried out in my laboratory during the past 20 years illustrate many of the principles involved in the production and modification of other specific appetites" (Richter 1956d, p. 378). Although he may not have been right about this, it illustrated what Richter and others understood as instinctive or innate behavior. Most of us in the field, myself included, would suggest that sodium is unique; there are few hard-wired ingestive systems such as the appetite for sodium (see Rozin and Schulkin 1990). But Richter, who contributed so much toward understanding ingestive behavior and the appetite for sodium in particular, led with his best intellectual punch.

Richter closed his talk with a discussion of the contrast between wild and domestic rats' regulatory and behavioral capacities. Even in this review of his work, Richter always stayed close to his data. He reveled in discussing his instruments and the rats' behavioral choices. The rootedness of the experiments in Richter's biological orientation to behavioral design was evident throughout the review. The one theoretical point that figured in his presentation was the concept of innate behavior, or what he called instinctive behavior.

In a conference packed with individuals who were theoretical by predilection and forthright in their criticism, Richter was methodological in his orientation (though grounded in the concept of instinct). After Richter noted an interesting observation about salt taste psychophysics and the putative role of the peripheral gustatory thresholds in several experiments, Lehrman asked Richter to comment on the psychophysical experiments demonstrating that rats that were not sodium hungry could discriminate salt as well as sodium-hungry rats could (e.g., Koh and Teitelbaum 1961). Lehrman cogently and, as it turned out, correctly asserted that "these data suggest that the effect of depletion may not be to changes in the sensitivity of the taste buds, but the role of salt as a reward." He continued, "in general, would you not agree that the experiments you describe are designed only to elucidate the facts of diet selection and its relationship to nutritional needs, and that the problem of the physiological and psychological mechanisms involved is still to a considerable extent an open one?" Richter briefly referred Lehrman to his first experiments with gustatory thresholds, saying, "The problems of the mechanisms underlying dietary self-selection are still unsettled, I quite agree." But he also said, "I would not agree that our experiments are designed only to elucidate facts of dietary selection and their relation to nutritional needs—certainly we try whenever possible to get an answer to the more fundamental problems of the underlying mechanisms" (Richter 1956d, p. 630). Another individual at the conference, J. Haldane, also queried Richter, saying that "I share Mr. Lehrman's skepticism on changing peripheral thresholds" (Richter 1956d, p. 630), as did a third attendee, H. Pierone (Richter 1956d, p. 631).

There were other queries after Richter's talk. One participant mentioned studies on African Pygmies in the forest and "the craving for salt by certain populations" (Richter 1956d, p. 629). Other investigators (J. Haldane, M. Klein) addressed the social value of salt. K. Von Frisch mentioned studies on the appetite for fat, suggesting that it is quite different from the appetite for salt as a model of appetitive behavior (Von Frisch 1956). M. Fontaine asked Richter how adrenalectomy and giving deoxycorticosterone could result in the same enhancement of salt ingestion. To this Richter replied, "To my knowledge we do not have an adequate explanation of these apparently opposing results" (Richter 1956d, p. 631).

Lehrman was concerned about the abuse of the concept of instinct and its potential misuse in understanding human motivation, creating false and misleading analogies between animals and humans. But there was a larger worry that goes back to the reification of the natural state.

Lehrman argued that Lorenz followed a line of thought in which the "effects of domestication" resulted in "the involution or degeneration of species-specific behavior patterns and releaser mechanisms because of degenerate mutations" (Lehrman 1953, p. 354). Lehrman criticized Lorenz for his flight into Nazi mythology and its destructive consequences (but see also Rosenblatt 1995). Richter does not seem to have been part of this conversation.

The nature versus nurture controversy had an intellectual paralyzing or polarizing effect then, as it does now. Richter tended to see everything "in the genes," even using the expression "the release of his genes" to depict his orientation. Richter believed that his work demonstrated the primacy of the biological point of view, but it was a laboratory, not a field, point of view.

World War II changed the intellectual landscape of the United States as well as of Europe. The concept of instinct, for some investigators, was tied to the eugenics espoused by the Nazis and their abuse of biological thought (Lehrman 1953). Many individuals were not entirely consistent in rejecting the concept of instinct, or at least a narrow notion of it (e.g., Lehrman 1954; Rosenblatt 1995). Still, there was legitimate concern about the abuse of the concept of instinct for behavioral explanations and about its vagueness as a scientifically meaningful construct. Frank Beach, in an interesting review titled "The Descent of Instinct," outlined the history of the concept of instinct from prescientific times to the modern period. Beach argued that the focus should be on the development of behavior and the stimuli that facilitate the behavioral expression of genes (Beach 1955). He believed that researchers should stay close to the behavioral analysis. Of course, Richter would be sympathetic to this.

In the field of ethology, Lorenz embraced ideological battles while Niko Tinbergen, who won a Nobel Prize with Lorenz, continued to reinforce and integrate various behavioral findings. Tinbergen's view was dominated by a common conception of the buildup of instinctive energy and its discharge in response to external stimuli. The greater the buildup, the more likely the discharge. Tinbergen suggested that "there are close parallels between the mechanisms underlying locomotion and that underlie an instinctive act" (Tinbergen 1951/1969, p. 71; see also Lorenz 1981). The nervous systems orchestrate the priorities of behavioral options. Tinbergen detailed the "reproductive instinct, and their hierarchical organization of behavior." He went on to suggest that "the various instincts are not independent of each other" (Tinbergen 1951/1969, p. 111). Although there was much discussion of innate systems in Tinbergen's work, there was very little discussion of learning. But Tinbergen did talk about motivational systems, a hierarchical organization of behavior that underlies instinctive behaviors (see also Thorpe 1948). W. H. Thorpe defined instinctive behaviors as comprising three features: inherited, specific, and stereotyped patterns of behavior (Thorpe 1948).

Both the internal buildup of drive and the configuration of external eliciting stimuli came to dominate ethological depictions of instinct (Lorenz 1981). Tinbergen published his book *The Study of Instinct* several years before the conference that he and Richter attended. In the book, Tinbergen carefully carved out the conceptual and experimental contexts for understanding the concept of instinct. As Tinbergen saw it, the motivation, or drive, aspect of instinctive behaviors is hydraulic in nature. The expression of instincts reflects both appetitive and consummatory behaviors (see also Craig 1918), and these behavioral features are hard-wired. Tinbergen emphasized rule-governed behavioral responses to specific sensory information. Instinct was embedded in this innate hardware, in terms of both the signals detected and the fixed action patterns emitted (Tinbergen 1951/1969).

Instinct and learning are inextricably linked, and although many ethologists emphasized fixed action patterns for the innate aspect of behaviors (Thorpe 1948) and motivational behaviors (Lashley 1938/1960; Stellar 1954), the concept of instinct can be tied to learning in which there is plasticity of expression (J. L. Gould 2002). An interesting array of prewired components are inherent in all behavior (Rozin 1976b). The question is how fixed and how flexible are the behavioral options? How easily can behavior be modified? We know from the strong link between gustatory information and visceral discomfort, for example, that stimuli are not of equal value (Garcia, Hankins, and Rusiniak 1974). In the concept of prepared learning, learning is steeped in innate factors and there is no rigid separation between what is innate and what is learned. Instinct is not on one side and learning on the other; many forms of learning are themselves instinctual.

Disparaging criticism of the stronghold of narrow behaviorism was leveled from many intellectual bastions, but perhaps the loudest and most ferocious came from ethologists. Lorenz and Tinbergen claimed that behaviorists "just don't know animals." This was a recurring theme in the autobiographical reminiscences of both Lorenz and Tinbergen (which, interestingly, appeared in the same volume as Richter's reflections). Ethologists were out to study behavior in the wild or to simulate the conditions of natural adaptation in the laboratory. They thought that innate hardware and built-up hydraulic drives converged to respond to specific configurations of external stimuli. Spontaneous behavior reflected the activation of hormones on central states of the brain (e.g., on motivational systems that underlie hunger). This is, of course, similar to Richter's ideas, minus his emphasis on biological clocks. There is little room for learning in this view. And that, I suggest, is a mistake, because innate predilection goes hand and hand with specialized forms of learning, adaptation, and multiple kinds of information processing, such as the phenomenon of human language (Pinker 1994).

Amid the raging debates on this concept of instinct and the legitimacy of psychology as a science, Richter went about generating experiments, taking the body apart and putting it back together again, and linking his research to broad-based behavioral and biological adaptation. He held to his data, his instruments, and his functionalistic explanations that bridged behavioral and physiological adaptation. He embraced Darwin, Bernard, and Cannon but understood the study of behavior as an engineer discerns the mechanisms that underlie adaptation. He was not part of the psychologists' search for the learning that underlies behavior.

RICHTER: FEARLESS AND FREE

Drawing on material he had presented to a committee at the National Research Council, Richter published an article in *Science* that drew heavily on his philosophical side. In this article, he advanced his views on what he called "free research versus design research." Richter stated his position clearly: "There is a choice before us between free and design research, or as I see it, between supporting the man or the experimental design" (Richter 1953f, p. 91). He shunned the modern culture of science that had evolved after World War II, having never really adapted to it. This was the culture of writing grants, of rigorous design in laying out one's plans. For Richter, this culture thwarted the process of investigation. He said, "We pick out the more tangible part of the application—the experimental design—how the man plans to work out his project." He worried greatly that by focusing almost exclusively on experimental design, science would lose sight of the researcher, and he felt that good researchers were being undermined. "It is not the design of the research," he said, "but the person, the individual scientist and their track record; one grant proposal may not reveal as much as the individual will, or one committee will not be able to know where it fits and what it will amount to." He went on to say that we must have faith in scientists and must recognize their past accomplishments: "The researcher has come to play a less and less important part; comparatively little is known about his background, setting, facilities, his sincerity [and his] determination and ability to carry on independent research. He is gradually being reduced to the status of a technician who must follow out in detail a definite plan of research" (Richter 1953f). For Richter, the individual gave validity to science, to experiment, and to a laboratory reproduction of ideas (see also Shapin and Schaffer 1985).

As the *Science* article illustrates, Richter was not of the era of experimental design. In later years, science would come to be dominated by statistics and design, but Richter had none of this. He explored in science. Discovery, he rightly understood, was based in part on what Kant (1790/1951) called the "free play of the imagination" and what Peirce called "abduction," or hitting on the right idea (Hanson 1971). Richter described a state of mind that involved "puzzlement of discrepancies in findings." This was, in fact, one condition for inquiry; inquiry often begins when discrepancies are noted (Peirce 1877). Modern learning theory is deeply tied to this view (Rescorla 1988). Richter also added another parenthetical remark, that "there are researchers who do not work on a verbal plane, who cannot put into words what they are doing" (Richter 1953f, p. 92). Richter, by his own account, thought not in terms of words or ideas, but instruments. He had what most interests investigators and artists: a capacity to play and to spend long periods puzzled, tinkering and discovering. There is no blueprint, no laid-out agenda in this approach. This is what he wanted protected and what he lamented as big science, in his view, lost track of the individual.

Richter captured a kernel of truth, but he was too steeped in a mythology that did not allow him to adapt to the burgeoning art of experimental design. In the *Science* article, he rightly recognized the importance of statistical design but asserted that it "should not substitute for ideas" (Richter 1953f, p. 92). Most of Richter's contemporaries, whatever their theoretical orientation, did not absorb statistical methods. An important contribution from behavioral psychology would be the logic of experimental design (e.g., the work of Neal Miller and Robert Rescorla). Experimental design would come to figure in all aspects of the behavioral sciences, as would the use of statistical analysis.

When Richter published the *Science* article, he was several years from emeritus status. He would continue doing research for another twenty-five years, but he was already behind the times. He was fortunate to have been supported in the way that he was. For example, some of his support came from the Rockefeller Foundation (1923–40, via Adolf Meyer), the National Institutes of Health (1952–65), the National Science Foundation (1956–77), the National Research Council (1937–45), the National Council on Alcoholism (1959–60), and the Commonwealth Fund (1964–77).

Richter probably always sought to escape the endless debates taking place within academic psychology. He remained a steadfast experimentalist, one who perhaps exaggerated innate behavioral solutions. He focused on the practical side of knowledge, the clinic, and patients. In these contexts, the engineer in Richter could come forward, extending and simplifying devices to measure physiological events that could be used to discern disease and dysfunction. Even at the very end of his life, Richter published papers on growth hormone (1980) and cortisol secretion (1983) in rats, guinea pigs, and monkeys and remained productive, active, and engaged in his scientific pursuits.

Epilogue

A week before Curt Richter died, I traveled to Baltimore with Paul Rozin and Jon Schull (a student of Rozin's, friend of mine, and then a teacher at Haverford College), to visit Richter. It would be the last visit. We three, in addition to many others, are inheritors of Richter's legacy. Even at that time, frail and soon to die, Richter was gracious and ready to interact with us. It was a short visit, but we left feeling warmed by his presence (fig. E.1). Richter had this effect on many people. He had a talent for it.

Guy McKhann, one of Richter's colleagues from the Neurology Department, remarked that Richter always seemed to be exploring or measuring something (G. McKhann, pers. comm., June 2003). And anyone who knew Richter understood that he was not afraid to explore. He lived in a culture that reinforced and cultivated his curiosity. Always, however, Richter was grounded in the practical and the physical. Guy McKhann recalled that when Richter needed to have a pacemaker implanted in his heart, he made sure it was inserted in such a way that it would not interfere with his tennis skill (G. McKhann, pers. comm., June 2003).

Richter had a quiet, reflective side, a side that perhaps did not always come forward. As he neared the end of his life, the biological basis of aging was on his mind. He kept notes on his own experience of aging, such as his loss of vision. When it was discovered that he had retinal detachment, he focused on the organization of the retina and visual acuity. As his friend McKhann noted, when Richter discovered an odd sensation in his finger or another part of his body, he was quick to begin inquiry into the phenomenon (G. McKhann, pers. comm., June 2003).

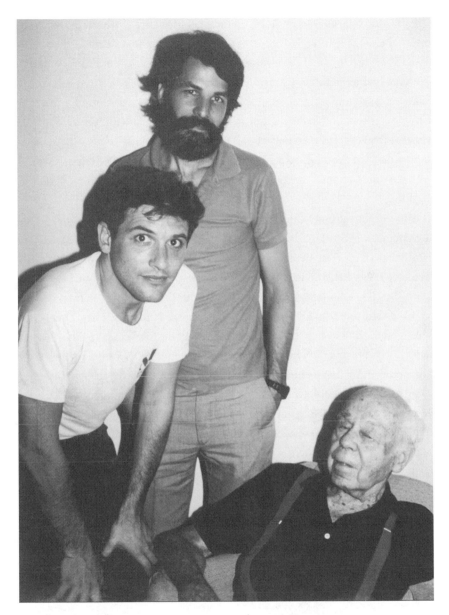

FIG. E.1. Two young assistant professors, Jon Schull *(standing)* and Jay Schulkin, with Richter shortly before his death in 1988. *Source:* Paul Rozin

Paul McHugh characterized Richter's relationship with Hopkins as "a union of assets" (McHugh 1989). At the start of his career, Richter had integrated well into the medical culture of that new school called Johns Hopkins. There he had encountered Adolf Meyer, whose views about total regulatory behavior, psychobiological adaptation, and clinical integration of a psychobiological orientation made legitimate what would become Richter's sixty-year career at the Hopkins medical school. A number of the colleagues and friends Richter made at the medical school (e.g., E. A. Park, head of pediatrics), would continue their connection with him over the duration of his long career at Hopkins.

Eliot Stellar wrote: "Curt Richer has been my model and inspiration for 50 years now" (Stellar files, University of Pennsylvania Archives). Stellar recalled that he first heard of Richter through his interaction with Cliff Morgan at Harvard, and Richter would remain close to Stellar until Richter's death. Stellar, who became the provost of the University of Pennsylvania, arranged for Richter to obtain a special degree from the university. He always looked on Richter as the "father of our field." Stellar was close to both Richter and his second wife, Leslie, and he wrote to her after Richter's death, "You know how much he meant to me. But I was only one of a whole generation of scientists he inspired" (Stellar files, University of Pennsylvania Archives, December 21, 1988). Hanging in Eliot Stellar's office was a tool Richter fashioned from an umbrella and heavy sock and used to inject and tube feed wild rats (fig. E.2).

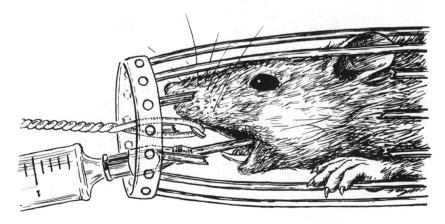

FIG. E.2. Part of an umbrella, used for injecting substances into wild rats. *Source:* Richter 1948c

Paul Rozin said much the same: "Curt is my model in many ways and represents an approach to science which I think I share" (P. Rozin, pers. comm., October 2003). I suspect this is not be an uncommon sentiment among investigators.

Elliott Blass captured the essence of Richter in this depiction of a meeting with him: "The incident occurred on a sunny fall day when Richter and I had an early morning appointment. I was walking along Wolfe Street towards Psychiatry and Curt was walking towards me, athletic, although a little frail. He was immaculately attired, as was his wont, in a gray suit sparkling white shirt and subdued tie and in his right hand was carrying a Have-A-Heart trap which contained a sprightly chipmunk. It all seemed so natural and contained all of the elements that embodied Curt" (E. Blass, pers. comm., October 2003).

Richter's influence, though selective, did cross the ocean. Derek Denton, from the University of Melbourne, recalled, "I first heard of Dr. Curt Richter's work when I was a medical student recently arrived in Melbourne from Tasmania in the mid-1940s. In those days, with communications as they were, and Australia relatively isolated, an important event was the occasional talk by a returned traveler telling what seemed novel and exciting in the outside scientific world" (Denton 1976, p. xxix). Denton heard of Richter from one of his colleagues and visited him on several occasions in Baltimore. Denton commented that "overall, in looking at the history of endocrinology during this century, it can be said that in the field of behavioral implications of internal secretions, Richter's contribution has been outstanding and the unique one" (Denton 1976).

STUBBORN AND TENACIOUS

Richter generated loyalty in those who worked with him and respect from those who understood his science, along with deep appreciation and wonder at the sheer scope of his investigations. It is said, however, that he could be extremely stubborn.

Richter's stubbornness remains legendary at Hopkins. Many people have related the story of trying to get Richter out of his laboratory space; he was very old but still holding on to the laboratory. Hopkins turned off the heat, and still he remained. Plaster peeled off the walls, and still he remained. The leaders of the Hopkins hospital sent over the young archivist Nancy McCall to coax him out with offers to help him with his papers. McCall was successful, in part because she offered to bring his work over to him and to care for his papers and his laboratory artifacts (N. McCall, pers. comm., August 2002).

Nancy McCall did more than implement the wishes of the Hopkins honchos by extracting Richter from his laboratory; she was truly helpful to Richter at the end of his life. She helped him submit his paper on Meyer to the *Journal of Behavioral Sciences.* The paper would have been published if Richter had agreed to make the apparently minor changes that the editor wanted, but Richter refused, so it never reached publication (McCall 1996; N. McCall, pers. comm., August 2002).

Richter's stubbornness in holding on to his laboratory may have reflected more than just a dogged personality. His papers and laboratory paraphernalia were a prop for him, a way to remain connected to his work and to his identity as a laboratory scientist (T. Moran, pers. comm., August 2002). Moreover, Richter continued to publish and mine the research and to write new papers, particularly about biological clocks, right up until the end of his life. His laboratory represented the paradigm of the laboratory state of mind for Richter, allowing him to stay within the culture of research.

C. S. Peirce emphasized the characteristic of tenacity in a scientist. It takes great tenacity to pursue one's scientific interests (Peirce 1877). The negative side of tenacity is to stubbornly hold onto a hypothesis or engage in a way of doing things even after it becomes unproductive. Richter, like all good scientists, suffered from the negative as well as benefited from the positive aspects of tenacity.

MINING THE DATA

Richter mined his own material throughout his lifetime. His laboratory books were neat and orderly, maintained by a devoted staff who took pride in contributing to science (A. O'Connor, pers. comm., July 2002). His laboratory notes reveal someone exploring, continuously jotting remarks about his subjects; periods of research interests are marked by sustained effort[1] (Moran and Schulkin 2000).

Richter was most productive in terms of publishing scientific papers from the 1930s through the 1950s. He managed to publish even in the 1920s when he was establishing his laboratory. In fact, there is no period in Richter's career, right from the beginning, when he was not scientifically productive. Richter stayed with core issues and experimental manipulations as he expanded into new terrain. He used his resources over and over again.

One does not get the sense that Richter changed his mind about core ideas; what would have made him think that perhaps a range of appetitive behaviors required various forms of learning? In fact, core ideas or metaphors underlie the behavior of all scientists (Galison 1988). For Richter, the core ideas centered around behavioral adaptation, regulation of the internal milieu, cyclic behavior, and instinctive behavior. Richter set out to demonstrate behavioral competence, the physiological signals that orchestrate adaptation to perturbations in the internal milieu.

A CAREER IN RESEARCH

Richter enjoyed considerable scientific success. Though less known than Cannon, Watson, and Lashley, he scaled to the heights of the American scientific establishment. Psychologists elected him to the most select scientific societies in the country, and he very much enjoyed participating in these prestigious societies.

It should not be surprising that Clifford Morgan dedicated the first edition of his book *Physiological Psychology* (Morgan 1943) to Lashley and Richter, two key people in psychobiological research. One was highly theoretical, the other thoroughly experimental. One dominated an intellectual culture, the other represented the paradigm of a laboratory state of mind. Lashley made fundamental contributions to the intellectual issues of the day and pushed the conceptual envelope; Richter continued to experiment and explore.

By the 1950s, a small but growing group of scientists devoted to understanding the regulation of specific hungers and circadian clocks within psychobiology would recognize the importance of Richter. During the 1950s, Richter was part of a group of investigators, including Pfaffmann, Young, Dethier, and Stellar, associated with setting standards for the preparation of solutions for research in ingestive behavior. Of these, Dethier, Richter, and Stellar were at Hopkins in three different departments: Psychology, Biology, and Psychiatry, respectively. Although many students of psychology might not recognize his name, there remains a large group of scientists all over the world who understand the importance of Richter to the field of psychobiology (Denton 1972, 1982). He was always understood as a serious investigator, serious enough to be nominated for the Nobel Prize and, on his death, to be described, along with Beach, Tinbergen, and Lorenz, as one of "four giants" (Dewsbury 1989).

Richter's contributions to the study of ingestive behavior have been catalogued by many investigators (e.g., Denton 1972; G. P. Smith 1997). In 1980, a conference on the biological and behavioral aspects of salt intake, at the Monell

Chemical Sense Center in Philadelphia, celebrated, in part, the research of Curt Richter (Kare, Fregly, and Bernard 1980).

I dedicated a book to Richter and started a series in honor of him, and several other individuals have dedicated papers and books to Richter. For example, Edward Stricker, a behavioral neuroscientist in the regulation of food and fluid intake and a student of Neal Miller, included the following dedication in his *Neurobiology of Food and Fluid Intake:* "This handbook is dedicated to the memory of Claude Bernard, Walter Cannon, and Curt Richter, whose pioneering work provided the foundation for the modern behavioral neurobiology of food and fluid intake" (Stricker 1990). There is the Curt Richter Prize for Outstanding Research, given by the journal *Psychoneuroendocrinology,* and there is the Curt Richter Chair in Chronobiology at Florida State University, currently held by Friedrich K. Stephans.

Richter continued to win awards, including the Passano Award in 1977, but to the place where he got his degree, he would remain largely a stranger, despite the fact that for several years Hopkins' Psychology Department had a Curt Richter lecture series (E. Blass, Stewart Hulse, P. Teitelbaum, and Howard Egeth, pers. comm., August 2000).

THE CLOSING OF RICHTER'S LABORATORY

I asked Timothy Moran, who has now been in Richter's department at Hopkins for close to thirty years and who knew Richter quite well, to tell me something about the closing of Richter's laboratory. Here is his response:

> Here is the story about the closure of Curt's lab. The lab was still in complete operation in 1975 when Paul McHugh became chair. In 1978–79, Paul and Curt came to the agreement that Curt's work with animals would stop. That part of the lab was closed and a part of it was converted to an ECT suite for the department. Bob Robinson was given Curt's running wheel cages and equipment for preparing the standard diet and used them until the late '80s. The Psychiatry Department moved out of the Phipps Clinic in the spring of 1982, except for the space occupied by Curt's lab and the small group environment laboratory that Joe Brady had established with NASA support. After about a year, renovation of the building began to convert the space for use by the School of Nursing. During that extensive renovation, there were times when there was no heat or air conditioning in the part of the building that Curt occupied. I don't remember the exact date that the lab closed but there was a small "celebration" to mark the event. By that time, the

building had been renovated except for Curt's space, and walking into Curt's lab was like going back in time. At the time of the move to the Meyer Building, Curt was offered space in the new building but declined since it was not sufficient space to bring along all his records. He also was offered space during the renovation, but again declined. The Institution was losing patience, as his space was wanted and the delay of closing the lab added significantly to the expense of renovating the building. However, they did allow him to remain through those years and the final closure was with his agreement (T. Moran, pers. comm., July 2003).

But it was a sad day, for Richter's life was embodied by that laboratory.

A CYBERCONFERENCE ON RICHTER

Chesney archivists Nancy McCall, Lisa Mix, and Marjorie Kehoe organized a cyberconference, inviting scholars to peruse and discuss Richter's archived documents. McCall and her colleagues at the archives broke new ground by looking to electronically preserve Richter's papers and notes. Their aim was to make Richter's material available to scientists and to generate interaction among them about this leader in the field of behavioral biology.

The cyberconference was introduced by Paul McHugh, Richter's last chairman and a great admirer of Richter. In his remarks, McHugh said that "Richter was a member of our faculty that we were most proud of here at Johns Hopkins, not only for the important research that he did, but particularly because of the way he did this research, systematically, coherently, and with data collection methods that were impeccable."

The cyberconference can be found on the Internet at www.medicalarchives .jhmi.edu/oldconfer/html/pbl/ricwelcm.htm. There one can read articles by Nancy McCall which lay out some of the history of Richter's laboratory. In "Richter's Long Farewell," a brief article about the closing of the laboratory, McCall notes that Richter wanted to reanalyze some of his data in light of new findings. In this and another article on the Web site, McCall also describes the archived documents and their condition, along with the interesting history of the documentation process.

The cyberconference Web site contains some outstanding articles about the contents of the Richter collection, a history of the Psychobiology Laboratory, possible data, interesting photographs, Watson's handwritten notes on the structure of the laboratory, and a bibliography of Richter. Other articles include two from students of Daniel Todes, a science historian of the behavioral sciences at Hopkins; one by Jesse Bump on Richter's general interests and another by Christine Keiner on the scientific structure of Richter's laboratory. Lisa Mix writes about the use of the Richter data collection, and Lynne Lamberg has included a piece about preserving the life of a laboratory. Lamberg also published an article in the *Journal of the American Medical Association* describing Richter and the cyberconference (Lamberg 1996).

RICHTER AND THE LABORATORY

Science is often discussed more in terms of the dominance of theory or observation than in terms of the interplay between theory, observation, and the instruments used in scientists' experimentation (see Galison 1987, 1988). Richter was rooted in some core ideas, but his reasoning focused on the experiment and laboratory invention and tools that aided the discovery of experimental facts.

As one colleague of Richter's insightfully characterized him: "Richter was more comfortable on the floor looking at the activity charts than discussing the ideas of the clocks and looking at people" (J. Wirth, pers. comm., September 2002). He is not known to a number of investigators and is often not mentioned in history textbooks when he should be (e.g., Finger 1994). But his legacy as a craftsman scientist will continue. He may not have been a good theorist, or cared to be. He was, however, a primary researcher who influenced a number of biologically oriented researchers, particularly after World War II.

Richter, unlike, for example, Cannon or Meyer, was not a public intellectual, nor did he cultivate a sense of what medical education should mean to students. Public intellectuals Cannon and Pavlov (see Todes 2002) nurtured many students who would become leaders in their fields. Richter's impact is often more circuitous. Many of us in the field, I would suggest, would consider ourselves students of Richter, not because we studied with him directly, but because of his influence on the field of psychobiology.

NOTES

1. The Flexner report was not without its critics (e.g., Berliner 1976; H. Miller 1966).

2. The Johns Hopkins model and the Flexner Report had a profound effect on medical education in the United States. The chair of my former department at the University of Pennsylvania was Louis Flexner. He, like his famous kin Abraham and Simon, understood that the laboratory and hands-on teaching were vital parts of medical school education. He lived to his nineties, maintaining an active laboratory.

1 ≡ ORIGINS AND ORIENTATIONS

1. Henderson's support of the experimental method no doubt influenced Richter, though I could find no mention of this influence other than a few passing remarks about Henderson in Richter's (1985) autobiography.

2. With regard to Dewey, Watson would recall how he "never knew what he was talking about" (Watson 1930/1961, p. 274). Watson would comment that he could barely understand the pragmatism that dominated the University of Chicago where he had been trained. He wanted something more rigorous than the pragmatism of John Dewey and George Herbert Mead. In Watson's mind, there was no room for what would later be characterized as a form of "cognitive behaviorism" (e.g., Tolman 1949). He preferred a radical behaviorism, a purge of talk about the mind. Dewey, for example, understood the new psychology, or psychobiology, as representing something open-ended, with cognitive adaptation as a primary feature. He saw behavioral adaptation, or self-corrective inquiry, as an essential part of our biology, our constitution (Dewey 1910/1965, 1925/1989). This is the form of classical pragmatism tied to American progressivism. The other side of pragmatism was tied to a narrower engineering perspective (cf. Schneider 1946/1963; J. E. Smith 1978; Pauly 1987; Weidman 1999; Dalton 2002).

3 ≡ INGESTIVE BEHAVIORS AND THE INTERNAL MILIEU

1. Bernard, like some other investigators, was formulating a philosophy in which science was conceived as part of the salvation of civilization. It was a purely materialistic

conception: no vitalism, no ghosts, just biological machinery that could be understood through experimental physiology and medicine (Holmes 1974, 2004).

2. Like his contemporary Pavlov and his predecessor Bernard, Starling was interested in pancreatic secretion, namely, the conditions under which chemicals are secreted for the digestion, absorption, and use of food sources (Bayliss and Starling 1902; see also Pavlov 1897/1902; G. P. Smith 2000; Todes 2002).

3. Anne Harrington, in a very interesting book on perceptual holism and its multiple meanings, depicts how the concept of instinct functioned in German science and cultural understanding (Harrington 1996). Richter stepped into a scientific world dominated by the concept of instinct and whether to retain or discard it. The central question about instinct was: What of behavior is innate and what is learned? But there were other discussions as well, such as to what extent the organization of behavior was a reflection of reflexes.

4 ≡ A PSYCHOBIOLOGICAL PERSPECTIVE ON THE DOMESTICATED AND THE WILD

1. See Logan's very thoughtful article on the use of and rationale for the rat as an experimental animal, and some of the confusion that surrounds the origins and justification of its use in this country (Logan 1999).

2. The experiments had a hygienic component—clearing the streets of Baltimore of vermin and disease—that was no doubt close to the heart of Adolf Meyer. After all, Meyer emphasized the hygienic aspects of diseases and health. Working with the mayor and the city council in a city where Richter had studied and worked for more than forty years was a broad application of his method of inquiry. Moreover, it had practical applications related to biological warfare and the country's defensive and offensive measures during a time of war and uncertainty.

3. Richter had a rugged sense about him; animals were to be trapped, examined, and used. After all, he noted that in his youth "coyote hunting constituted a rare but exciting pleasure" (Richter 1985, p. 360). He held no romanticism about animals; he might appreciate their utility, but he had no appreciation of their inherent beauty. Richter hailed from the wild (or near-wild) West. In Colorado at the turn of the twentieth century, one captured, ate, and (in his own case) studied animals, and perhaps one had a few pets.

4. See Kohler 2002 for a discussion of the tension between what one produces in the laboratory and what one observes in nature, and between the laboratory scientist and the more ethological or ecological scientist.

EPILOGUE

1. See Holmes for a discussion of tracing laboratory notes and empirical or experimental results for Claude Bernard (Holmes 1974) and Hans Krebs (Holmes 1993).

REFERENCES

Note: For works of which Curt P. Richter was author or coauthor, see the bibliography that follows.

Andrus, E. C., D. W. Bronk, G. A. Carden Jr., C. S. Keefer, J. S. Lockwood, J. T. Wearn, and M. D. Winternitz, eds. 1948. *Advances in Military Medicine.* Boston: Little, Brown.

Angell, J. R., et al. 1896. *Studies from the Psychological Laboratory: The University of Chicago Contributions to Philosophy.* Chicago: University of Chicago Press.

Aschoff, J. 1981. Biological rhythms. *Handbook of Behavioral Neurobiology,* vol. 4. New York: Plenum Press.

Aschoff, J., and R. Wever. 1965. Circadian rhythms of finches in light dark cycles with interposed twilights. *Comparative Biochemistry and Physiology* 16:507–14.

Aschoff, J., U. Gerecke, and R. Wever. 1967. Desynchronization of human circadian rhythms. *Journal of General Physiology* 17:450–57.

Barbour, T. 1943. *Naturalist at Large.* Boston: Little, Brown.

Barnett, S. A. 1956. Behaviour components in the feeding of wild and laboratory rats. *Behaviour* 9:24–43.

———. 1963. *The Rat: A Study in Behaviour.* Chicago: Aldine.

Bartoshuk, L. 1974. NaCl thresholds in man: Thresholds for water taste or NaCl taste. *Journal of Comparative and Physiological Psychology* 87:310–25.

Bauer, M., A. Heinz, and P. C. Whybrow. 2002. Thyroid hormones, serotonin and mood: Of synergy and significance in the adult brain. *Molecular Psychiatry* 7:140–56.

Bayliss, W. M., and E. H. Starling. 1902. The mechanisms of pancreatic secretion. *Journal of Physiology* 28:325–55.

Bazett, H. G., and W. G. Penfield. 1922. A study of the Sherrington decerebrate animal in the chronic as well as the acute condition. *Brain* 45:185–97.

Beach, F. A. 1955. The descent of instinct. *Psychological Review* 62:401–10.

Beer, C. G. 1983. Darwin, instinct and ethology. *Journal of the History of the Behavioral Sciences* 19:68–80.

Benison, S., A. C. Barger, and E. L. Wolfe. 1987. *Walter B. Cannon: The Life and Times of a Young Scientist.* Cambridge: Harvard University Press.

Benjamin, L. T. 1988. *A History of Psychology.* New York: McGraw Hill.

Berliner, H. S. 1976. A larger perspective on the Flexner Report. *International Journal of Health Services* 5:573–92.

Bernard, C. 1856/1985. *Memoir on the Pancreas.* New York: Academic Press.

———. 1865/1957. *An Introduction to the Study of Experimental Medicine.* New York: Dover Press.

Blass, E. M., ed. 1976. *The Psychobiology of Curt Richter.* Baltimore: York Press.

Boakes, R. 1984. *From Darwin to Behaviourism.* Cambridge: Cambridge University Press.

Boice, R. 1973. Domestication. *Psychological Bulletin* 80:215–30.

Boring, E. G. 1929/1950. *History of Experimental Psychology.* New York: Appleton-Century-Crofts.

Brendt, J. 1993. *C. S. Peirce: A Life.* Bloomington: Indiana University Press.

Broca, P. 1861/1960. Remarks on the seat of the faculty of articulate language. In *Some Papers of the Cerebral Cortex,* edited by G. Von Bonin. Springfield, Ill.: Charles C. Thomas.

Brödel, M. 1941. Medical illustration. *JAMA* 117:668–72.

———. 1946. *Three Unpublished Drawings of the Anatomy of the Human Ear.* Philadelphia: W. B. Saunders.

Buckley, K. W. 1989. *Mechanical Man: J. B. Watson and the Beginnings of Behaviorism.* New York: Guilford Press.

Bump, J. B. 1996. Arts of resistance, myths of reference: Curt Richter's skin resistance testing and the U.S. Army. Unpublished manuscript.

Bunning, E. 1963. *Die Physiologische Uhr,* 2nd ed. Berlin: Springer.

Cadwallader, T. C. 1974. Charles S. Peirce (1839–1914): The first American experimental psychologist. *Journal of the History of the Behavioral Sciences* 10:291–98.

Cannon, W. B. 1915/1929. *Bodily Changes in Pain, Hunger, Fear and Rage.* New York: Harper & Row.

———. 1932/1966. *The Wisdom of the Body.* New York: Norton Press.

———. 1942. Voodoo death. *American Anthropologist* 44:169–81.

Carlson, A. J. 1916. *The Control of Hunger in Health and Disease.* Chicago: University of Chicago Press.

Cetina, K. K. 1999. *Epistemic Culture.* Cambridge: Harvard University Press.

Chapman, F. M. 1938. *Life in an Air Castle: Nature Studies in the Tropics.* New York: D. Appleton-Century.

Chesney, A. M. 1943–63. *The Johns Hopkins Hospital and the Johns Hopkins University School of Medicine,* vols. 1–3. Baltimore: Johns Hopkins Press.

Collier, G., and D. F. Johnson. 1997. Who is in charge? Animal vs. experimenter control. *Appetite* 29:159–80.

Contreras, R. J. 1977. Changes in gustatory nerve discharges with sodium deficiency: A single unit analysis. *Brain Research* 121:343–48.

Craig, W. 1918. Appetites and aversions as constituents of instincts. *Biological Bulletin* 34:96–103.

Critchley, M., and E. A. Critchley. 1998. *John Hughlings Jackson: Father of English Neurology.* Oxford: Oxford University Press.

Crosby, R. W., and J. Cody. 1991. *Max Brodel: The Man Who Put Art into Medicine.* New York: Springer-Verlag.

Cross, S. J., and W. R. Albury. 1987. Walter B. Cannon, L. J. Henderson, and the organic analogy. *ORISIS* 3:165–92.

Crowe, S. J. 1957. *Halsted of Johns Hopkins.* Springfield, Ill.: Charles C. Thomas.

Cullen, T. S. 1945. Max Brodel, 1870–1941, director of the first Department of Art as Applied to Medicine in the world. *Bulletin of the Medical Library Association* 33: 5–28.

Dalton, T. C. 2002. *Becoming John Dewey: Dilemmas of a Philosopher and Naturalist.* Bloomington: Indiana University Press.

Darwin, C. 1859/1965. *The Origin of Species.* New York: Mentor Books.

———. 1868/1892. *Variation of Animals and Plants under Domestication,* vols. 1 and 2. New York: Appleton.

———. 1871/1874. *The Descent of Man and Selection in Relation to Sex.* Chicago: Rand McNally.

———. 1872/1998. *The Expression of the Emotions in Man and Animals.* Oxford: Oxford University Press.

———. 1873. Inherited instinct. *Nature* 7:281–85.

da Vinci, L. 1980. *The Notebooks,* edited by I. A. Richter. Oxford: Oxford University Press.

Davis, C. 1928. Self-selection of diets by newly weaned infants: An experimental study. *American Journal of Diseases of Children* 36:651–79.

———. 1935. Self-selection of food by children. *American Journal of Nursing* 35:402–10.

———. 1939. Results of the self-selection of diets by young children. *Canadian Medical Association Journal* 41:257–61.

Denton, D. A. 1972. Instinct, appetites and medicine. *Australia and New Zealand Journal of Medicine* 2:203–12.

———. 1976. Tribute to Curt Richter. In *The Psychobiology of Curt Richter,* edited by E. M. Blass. Baltimore: York Press.

———. 1982. *The Hunger for Salt.* Berlin: Springer-Verlag.

Dethier, V. G. 1976. *The Hungry Fly.* Cambridge: Harvard University Press.

Dewey, J. 1910/1965. *The Influence of Darwin on Philosophy.* Bloomington: Indiana University Press.

———. 1916. *Essays in Experimental Logic.* New York: Dover Press.

———. 1925/1989. *Experience and Nature.* LaSalle, Ill.: Open Court Press.

———. 1934/1958. *Art as Experience.* New York: Capricorn Books.

Dewsbury, D. A. 1989. Four giants: Frank Beach, Curt Richter, Niko Tinbergen and Konrad Lorenz. *Animal Behavioral Society* 34:1–3.

————. 1991. Psychobiology. *American Psychologist* March, 198–205.

————. 1992. William James and instinct theory revisited. In *Reinterpreting the Legacy of William James*, edited by M. E. Donnelly. Washington, D.C.: American Psychological Association.

Donaldson, H. H. 1915. The rat data and reference tables for the albino and the Norway rat. *Memoirs of the Wistar Institute of Anatomy and Biology*, no. 6. Philadelphia: Wistar Institute.

Dove, W. F. 1935. A study of individuality in the nutritive instincts and of the causes and effects of variations in the selection of food. *American Naturalist* 69:469–544.

Dunlap, K. 1914. *An Outline of Psychobiology*. Baltimore: Johns Hopkins Press.

————. 1919. Are there any instincts? *Journal of Abnormal Psychology* 14:307–11.

Epstein, A. N. 1982. Instinct and motivation as explanations for complex behavior. In *The Physiological Mechanisms of Motivation*, edited by D. Pfaff, 25–55. New York: Springer-Verlag.

Epstein, A. N., and E. Stellar. 1955. The control of salt preference in the adrenalectomized rat. *Journal of Comparative and Physiological Psychology* 48:167–72.

Evvard, J. M. 1915. Is the appetite of swine a reliable indication of physiological need? *Proceedings of the Iowa Academy of Science* 22:375–402.

Finger, S. 1994. *Origins of Neuroscience*. Oxford: Oxford University Press.

Fitzsimons, J. T. 1979. *The Physiology of Thirst and Sodium Appetite*. Cambridge: Cambridge University Press.

Flexner, A. 1910/1978. *Medical Education in the United States and Canada*. Boston: D. B. Updike, The Merrymount Press.

Freud, S. 1920/1975. *Beyond the Pleasure Principle*. New York: W. W. Norton.

Friedman, M. I., I. Ramirez, N. K. Edens, and J. Granneman. 1985. Food intake in diabetic rats: isolation of primary metabolic effects of fat feeding. *American Journal of Physiology* 249:R44–51.

Frumovitz, M. M. 2002. Thomas Eakins' Agnew Clinic: A study of medicine through art. *Obstetrics and Gynecology* 100:1296–300.

Galef, B. G., Jr. 1991. A contrarian view of the wisdom of the body as it relates to dietary self-selection. *Psychological Review* 98:218–23.

Galef, B. G., Jr. and E. E. Whiskin. 2001. Effects of caloric, protein and sodium deprivation on the affiliative behavior of Norway rats. *Journal of Comparative Physiology* 115:192–95.

Galison, P. 1987. *How Experiments End*. Chicago: University of Chicago Press.

————. 1988. History, philosophy and the central metaphor. *Science in Context* 3:197–212.

Garcia, J., W. G. Hankins, and K. W. Rusiniak. 1974. Behavioral regulation of the milieu interne in man and rat. *Science* 185:824–31.

Gilman, D. C. 1906. *The Launching of a University and Other Papers*. New York: Dodd Mead.

Gould, J. L. 2002. Learning instincts. In *Steven's Handbook of Experimental Psychology*, 3rd ed., edited by H. Pashler and R. J. Gallistel, 3:239–57. New York: John Wiley & Sons.

Gould, S. J. 2002. *The Structure of Evolutionary Theory*. Cambridge: Harvard University Press.

Grasse, P. P., ed. 1956. *L'instinct dans le comportement des animaux et de l'homme*. Paris: Masson et Cie Editeurs.

Green, H. H. 1925. Perverted appetites. *Physiology Review* 5:336–48.

Grifiths, W. J. 1960. Responses of wild and domestic rats to forced swimming. *Psychological Reports* 6:39–49.

Grill, H. J., and R. Norgren. 1978. The taste reactivity test II: Mimetic responses to gustatory stimuli in chronic thalamic and chronic decerebrate rats. *Brain Research* 100: 536–43.

Hall, C. V. 1941. Temperament: A survey of animal studies. *Psychological Bulletin* 38:909–43.

Hanson, N. R. 1971. *Observation and Explanation*. New York: Harper Torchbooks.

Harrington, A. 1996. *Re-enchanted Science: Holism in German Culture from Wilhelm II to Hitler*. Princeton, N.J.: Princeton University Press.

Harris, L. J., J. Clay, F. Hargreaves, and A. Ward. 1933. Appetite and choice of diet: The ability of the vitamin B deficient rat to discriminate between diets containing and lacking the vitamin. *Proceedings of the Royal Society of London*, series B, 113:161–90.

Harvey, A. M., G. H. Brieger, S. L. Abrams, and V. A. McKusick. 1989. *A Centennial History of Medicine at Johns Hopkins*, vol. 1. Baltimore: Johns Hopkins University Press.

Hawkins, H. 1960. *Pioneer: A History of the Johns Hopkins University, 1874–1889*. Ithaca, N.Y.: Cornell University Press.

Hebb, D. O. 1949. *The Organization of Behavior*. New York: John Wiley & Sons.

Helmholtz, H. 1867/1963. *Handbook of Physiological Optics*. New York: Dover Press.

Henderson, L. J. 1935. The relation of medicine to the fundamental sciences. *Science* 82:477–81.

———. 1970. *Selected Writings*, edited by B. Barber. Chicago: University of Chicago Press.

Herrnstein, R. J. 1972. Nature as nurture: Behaviorism and the instinct doctrine. *Behaviorism* 1:23–52.

Hess, E. H. 1973. *Imprinting*. New York: Van Nostrand Reinhold.

Hilgard, E. R. 1987. *Psychology in America*. New York: Harcourt Brace Jovanovich.

Hollinger, D. A. 1994. The knower and the artificer. In *Modernist Impulses in the Human Sciences, 1870–1930*, edited by D. Ross. Baltimore: Johns Hopkins University Press.

Holmes, F. L. 1974. *Claude Bernard and Animal Chemistry*. Cambridge: Harvard University Press.

———. 1993. *Hans Krebs: Architect of Intermediary Metabolism*, vol. 2. Oxford: Oxford University Press.

————. 2004. *Investigative Pathways*. New Haven, Conn.: Yale University Press.

Holt, E. B. 1915. *The Freudian Wish and Its Place in Ethics*. New York: Henry Holt.

————. 1931/1976. *Animal Drive and the Learning Process: An Essay toward Radical Empiricism*. New York: Octagon Books.

————. 1937. Materialism and the criterion of the psychic. *Psychological Review* 44: 35–53.

Hudson, R. P. 1972. Abraham Flexner in perspective. *Bulletin of the History of Medicine* 46:545–61.

Hughes, C. W., and J. J. Lynch. 1978. A reconsideration of psychological precursors of sudden death in infrahuman animals. *American Psychologist* May, 419–29.

Hull, C. L. 1943. *Principles of Behavior*. New York: Appleton-Century-Crofts.

Jackson, H. 1884/1958. Evolution and dissolution of the nervous system. In *Selected Writings of John Hughlings Jackson*, edited by J. Taylor. London: Staples Press.

James, W. 1887. What is an instinct? *Scribners Magazine* 1:355–65.

————. 1890/1952. *The Principles of Psychology*. New York: Dover Press.

————. 1907/1958. *Pragmatism*. New York: Meridian Books.

————. 1907/1968. The energies of men. In *The Writings of William James*. New York: Modern Library.

Jennings, H. S. 1907. The interpretation of the behavior of lower organisms. *Science* 27:698–710.

Johnson, M. S. 1926. Activity and distribution of certain mice in relation to biotic communities. *Journal of Mammalogy* 245–77.

Kagan, J. 1989. *Unstable Ideas*. Cambridge: Harvard University Press.

Kant, I. 1790/1951. *Critique of Judgment*. New York: Bobbs-Merrill.

Kare, M. R., M. J. K. Fregly, and R. A. Bernard, eds. 1980. *Biological and Behavioral Aspects of Salt Intake*. New York: Academic Press.

Keiner, C. M. 1996. Social and scientific organization in the Psychobiology Laboratory, 1935–1978. First International Conference on the Psychobiology of Curt P. Richter.

Kinder, E. F. 1927. A study of the nest building activity of the albino rat. *Journal of Experimental Zoology* 47:117–61.

King, H. D. 1930. Life processes in gray Norway rats during fourteen years in captivity. *American Anatomical Memoirs* 17:1–72.

King, H. D., and H. H. Donaldson. 1929. Life processes and size of the body and organs of the gray Norway rat during ten generations in captivity. *American Anatomical Memoirs* 14:1–106.

Kissileff, H. R., and A. N. Epstein. 1969. Exaggerated prandial drinking in the recovered lateral rat with saliva. *Journal of Comparative and Physiological Psychology* 67: 301–8.

Klerman, G. 1979. The psychology of affective states: The legacy of Adolf Meyer. In *Research in the Psychobiology of Human Behavior*, edited by E. Meyer III and J. V. Brady. Baltimore: Johns Hopkins University Press.

Koh, S. D., and P. Teitelbaum. 1961. Absolute behavioral taste thresholds in the rat. *Journal of Comparative and Physiological Psychology* 54:223–29.

Kohler, R. E. 1991. *Partners in Science.* Chicago: University of Chicago Press.

———. 2002. *Landscapes and Laboratories.* Chicago: University of Chicago Press.

Kon, S. K. 1931. The self-selection of food constituents by the rat. *Biochemical Journal* 25:473–81.

Kuhn, T. S. 1962. *The Structure of Scientific Revolution.* Chicago: University of Chicago Press.

Lamberg, L. 1996. Cyber-conference helps archivists manage trove of scientific papers. *JAMA* 276:1935–37.

Lashley, K. S. 1938/1960. Experimental analysis of instinctive behavior. In *The Neuropsychology of Lashley*, edited by F. A. Beach, D. O. Hebb, C. L. Morgan, and H. W. Nissen, chap. 23. New York: McGraw Hill.

Lashley, K. S., and J. B. Watson. 1913. Notes on the development of a young monkey. *Journal of Animal Behavior* 3:114–39.

Lat, J. 1967. Self-selection of dietary components. In *Handbook of Physiology*, sect. 6, *Alimentary Canal*, vol. 1, *Control of Food and Water Intake*, edited by C. F. Code, 367–86. Washington, D.C.: American Physiological Society.

Latour, B., and S. Woolgar. 1979/1986. *Laboratory Life.* Princeton, N.J.: Princeton University Press.

Lehrman, D. S. 1953. A critique of Konrad Lorenz's theory of instinctive behavior. *Quarterly Review of Biology* 28(4):337–63.

———. 1954. Parental behavior in birds and the problem of "instinct." *Acta Psychologica* 11:96–97.

———. 1956. On the organization of maternal behavior and the problem of instinct. In *L'instinct dans le comportement des animaux et de l'homme*, edited by P. P. Grasse, chap. 13. Paris: Masson et Cie Editeurs.

Leigh, E. G. 1999. *Tropical Forest Ecology.* Oxford: Oxford University Press.

Leshem, M., S. Delcancho, and J. Schulkin. 1999. Ontogeny of calcium preference in the parathyroidectomized rat. *Developmental Psychobiology* 34:293–301.

Leys, R. 1984. Meyer, Watson, and the dangers of behaviorism. *Journal of the History of the Behavioral Sciences* 20:128–49.

Leys, R., and R. B. Evans. 1990. *Defining American Psychology: The Correspondence between Adolf Meyer and Edward Titchener.* Baltimore: Johns Hopkins University Press.

Liddell, E. G. T., and C. Sherrington. 1924. Reflexes in response to stretch (myostatic reflexes). *Proceedings of the Royal Society of London*, series B, 90:212–43.

Lidz, T. 1966. Adolf Meyer and the development of American psychiatry. *American Journal of Psychiatry* 123(3):320–32.

Loeb, J. 1918/1973. *Forced Movements, Tropisms and Animal Conduct.* New York: Dover Press.

Logan, C. A. 1999. The altered rationale for the choice of a standard animal in experimental psychology: Henry H. Donaldson, Adolf Meyer and the albino rat. *History of Psychology* 2:3–24.

Lorenz, K. 1956. The objectivistic theory of instinct. In *L'instinct dans le comportement des animaux et de l'homme*, edited by P. P. Grasse, chap. 3. Paris: Masson et Cie Editeurs.

———. 1981. *The Foundations of Ethology*. New York: Simon & Schuster.

Lynch, M. 1985. *Art and Artifact in Laboratory Science*. London: Routledge & Kegan Paul.

McCall, N. 1996. A brief history of the psychobiology laboratory. First International Cyberconference on the Psychobiology of Curt P. Richter.

McCollum, E. V. 1964. *From Kansas Farm Boy to Scientist*. Lawrence: University of Kansas Press.

McCollum, E. V., N. Simmonds, M. Kinney, P. G. Shipley, and E. A. Park. 1922. Studies on experimental rickets, XVII. *American Journal of Hygiene* 2(2):280–89.

McDougall, W. 1910. *An Introduction to Social Psychology*, 3rd ed. Boston: J. W. Luce.

McEachron, D. L., and J. Schull. 1993. Hormones, rhythms and the blues. In *Hormonally Induced Changes in Mind and Brain*, edited by J. Schulkin. New York: Academic Press.

McHugh, P. R. 1989. Curt Richter and Johns Hopkins: A union of assets. *American Journal of Physiology* 256:169–70.

McHugh, P. R., and P. R. Slavney. 1998. *The Perspectives of Psychiatry*, 2nd ed. Baltimore: Johns Hopkins University Press.

Meyer, A. 1915. Objective psychology or psychobiology with subordination of the medically useless contrast of mental and physical. *JAMA* 65:860–63.

———. 1931/1957. *Psychobiology*. Springfield, Ill.: Charles C. Thomas.

———. 1935. Scope and teaching of psychobiology. *JAMA* 10:93–98.

———. 1951. *The Collected Papers of Adolf Meyer*, edited by E. E. Winters. 4 vols. Baltimore: Johns Hopkins Press.

Miller, H. 1966. Fifty years after Flexner. *Lancet* 11:647–54.

Miller, N. E. 1979. Psychosomatic effects of learning. In *Research in the Psychobiology of Human Behavior*, edited by E. Meyer III and J. V. Brady. Baltimore: Johns Hopkins University Press.

Moore, R. Y., and V. B. Eichler. 1972. Loss of a circadian adrenal corticosterone rhythm following suprachiasmatic lesions in the rat. *Brain Research* 42:201–6.

Moran, T. H., and J. Schulkin. 2000. Curt Richter and regulatory physiology. *American Journal of Physiology* 279:R357–63.

Morgan, C. L. 1910. Instinct and intelligence. *British Journal of Psychology* 3:219–29.

Morgan, C. T. 1943. *Physiological Psychology*. New York: McGraw Hill.

Morgan, C. T., and E. Stellar. 1950. *Physiological Psychology*, 2nd ed. New York: McGraw Hill.

Morin, L. P., K. M. Fitzgerald, and I. Zucker. 1977. Estradiol shortens the period of hamster circadian rhythms. *Science* 196:305–7.

Mrosovsky, N., and D. Janik. 1993. Behavioral decoupling of circadian rhythms. *Journal of Biological Rhythms* 8:57–65.

Nachman, M. 1962. Taste preferences for sodium salts by adrenalectomized rats. *Journal of Comparative and Physiological Psychology* 55:1124–29.

Nelson, R. J. 1995. *An Introduction to Behavioral Endocrinology*. Sunderland, Mass.: Sinauer Associates.

Numbers, R. L., and C. E. Rosenberg, eds. 1996. *The Scientific Enterprise in America*. Chicago: University of Chicago Press.

O'Donnell, J. M. 1985. *The Origins of Behaviorism*. New York: New York University Press.

Olmsted, J. M. D. 1944. *Francois Magendie, Pioneer in Experimental Physiology and Scientific Medicine in XIX Century France*. New York: Schuman's.

Olmsted, J. M. D., and E. H. Olmsted. 1952. *Claude Bernard and the Experimental Method in Medicine*. New York: Henry Schuman.

Ormsbee, R. A. 1948. The development of new rodenticides. In *Advances in Military Medicine*. Boston: Little, Brown.

Osborne, T. B., and L. B. Mendel. 1918. The choice between adequate and inadequate diets, as made by rats. *Journal of Biological Chemistry* 35:19–27.

Pauly, P. J. 1979. Psychology at Hopkins. *Johns Hopkins Magazine* 30:36–41.

———. 1987. *Controlling Life*: *Jacques Loeb and the Engineering Ideal in Biology*. Oxford: Oxford University Press.

Pavlov, I. P. 1897/1902. *Lectures on the Work of the Digestive Glands*, translated by W. H. Thompson. London: Charles Griffin.

———. 1941/1967. *Lectures on Conditioned Reflexes*, vol. 2, *Conditioned Reflexes and Psychiatry*, translated and edited by W. H. Gantt. New York: International.

Peirce, C. S. 1877. The fixation of belief. *Popular Scientific Monthly* 12:1–15.

———. 1878. How to make our ideas clear. *Popular Scientific Monthly* 18:286–302.

———. 1898/1992. *Reasoning and the Logic of Things*. Cambridge: Harvard University Press.

Perry, R. B. 1935. *The Thought and Character of William James*. Boston: Little, Brown.

Pfaffmann, C. 1967. The sense of taste. In *Handbook of Physiology*, sect. 6, *Alimentary Canal*, vol. 1, *Control of Food and Water Intake*, edited by C. F. Code. Washington, D.C.: American Physiological Society.

Pinker, S. 1994. *The Language Instinct*. New York: William Morrow.

Pittendrigh, C. S. 1974. Circadian oscillations in cells and the circadian organization of multicellular systems. In *The Neurosciences*: *Third Study Program*, edited by F. O. Schmitt and F. G. Worden, 437–58. Cambridge, Mass.: MIT Press.

Prendergast, B. J., R. J. Nelson, and I. Zucker. 2002. Mammalian seasonal rhythms: Behavior and neuroendocrine substrates. In *Hormones, Brain and Behavior*, vol. 2., edited by D. W. Pfaff, A. P. Arnold, A. M. Etgen, S. E. Fahrbach, and R. T. Rubin. New York: Academic Press.

Prentice, A. 1994. Maternal calcium requirements during pregnancy and lactation. *American Journal of Clinical Nutrition* 59:477–83.

Price, E. O. 1984. Animal domestication. *Quarterly Review of Biology* 59:1–32.

———. 2002. *Animal Domestication and Behavior*. Oxford: CABI/Oxford University Press.

Rescorla, R. A. 1988. Pavlovian conditioning: It's not what you think it is. *American Psychologist* 45:151–60.

Roe, A. 1953. *The Making of a Scientist*. New York: Dodd Mead.

Roland, N. E., and M. J. Fregly. 1988. Sodium appetite: species and strain differences in the induction of sodium appetite: role of rennin-angiotensin-aldosterone system. *Appetite* 11:143–78.

Rosenberg, C. E. 1976/1997. *No Other Gods*. Chicago: University of Chicago Press.

Rosenblatt, J. S. 1995. *Daniel Sanford Lehrman, June 1, 1919–August 27, 1972*. Washington, D.C.: National Academy Press.

Rosenwasser, A. M., and N. T. Adler. 1986. Structure and function in circadian timing systems: Evidence for multiple coupled circadian oscillators. *Neuroscience and Biobehavioral Reviews* 10:431–48.

Rosenzweig, M. R., and E. L. Bennett. 1996. Psychobiology of plasticity: Effects of training and experience on brain and behavior. *Behavioral Brain Research* 78:57–65.

Rozin, P. 1967. Thiamine specific hunger. In *Handbook of Physiology*, sect. 6, *Alimentary Canal*, vol. 1, *Control of Food and Water Intake*, edited by C. F. Code, 411–32. Washington, D.C.: American Physiological Society.

———. 1976a. The compleat psychobiologist. In *The Psychobiology of Curt Richter*, edited by E. M. Blass. Baltimore: York Press.

———. 1976b. The selection of foods by rats, humans, and other animals. In *Advances in the Study of Behavior*, vol. 6, edited by J. Rosenblatt, R. A. Hinde, C. Beer, and E. Shaw, 21–76. New York: Academic Press.

Rozin, P., and J. W. Kalat. 1971. Specific hungers and poison avoidance as adaptive specialization of learning. *Psychological Review* 78:459–86.

Rozin, P., and J. Schulkin. 1990. Food selection. In *Handbook of Behavioral Neurobiology*, edited by E. M. Stricker. New York: Plenum Press.

Rusak, B. 2000. Chronobiology and mood disorders: background and introduction. *Journal of Psychiatry and Neuroscience* 25(5):443–44.

Rusak, B., and I. Zucker. 1979. Neural regulation of circadian rhythms. *Physiological Reviews* 59:449–526.

Sadovnikova-Koltzova, M. P. 1926. Genetic analysis of temperament of rats. *Journal of Experimental Zoology* 45:301–18.

Schneider, H. W. 1946/1963. *A History of American Philosophy*. New York: Columbia University Press.

Schneirla, T. C. 1956. Interrelationships of the "innate" and the "acquired" in instinctive behavior. In *L'instinct dans le comportment des animaux*, edited by P. P. Grasse, 387–452. Paris: Masson et Cie Editeurs.

Schulkin, J. 1978. Mineralocorticoids, dietary conditions and sodium appetite. *Behavioral Biology* 23:197–205.

———. 1989. In honor of a great inquirer: Curt Richter. *Psychobiology* 17:113–14.

———. 1991. *Sodium Hunger.* Cambridge: Cambridge University Press.

Schulkin, J., P. Rozin, and E. Stellar. 1994. *Curt Richter: Biographical Memoirs.* Washington, D.C.: National Academy of Sciences Press 65:311–20.

Schultheiss, D., and U. Jonas. 1999. Max Brodel and Howard A. Kelley: Urogynecology and the birth of modern medical illustration. *European Journal of Obstetrics and Gynecology and Reproductive Biology* 86:113–15.

Scott, E. M. 1946. Self selection of diet. 1. Selection of purified components. *Journal of Nutrition* 31:497–405.

Scott, E. M., and E. L. Verney. 1949. Self selection of diet: The appetite for thiamine. *Journal of Nutrition* 37:81–91.

Seligman, M. E. P. 1972. Learned helplessness. *Annual Review of Medicine* 23:407–11.

Selye, H. 1946. The general adaptation syndrome and the diseases of adaptation. *Journal of Clinical Endocrinology* 6:117–46.

Shapin, S. 1989. The invisible technician. *American Scientist* 77:534–63.

Shapin, S., and S. Schaffer. 1985. *Leviathan and the Air-Pump.* Princeton, N. J.: Princeton University Press.

Shettleworth, S. J. 1972. Constraints on learning. In *Advances in the Study of Behavior,* vol. 4, edited by D. S. Lehrman, R. A. Hinde, and F. Shaw, 1–68. New York: Academic Press.

Smith, G. P. 1989. Remarks at a Memorial Meeting for Curt Richter at the Department of Psychiatry, Johns Hopkins Medical School.

———. 1997. Eating and the American Zeitgeist. *Appetite* 29:191–200.

———. 2000. Pavlov and integrative physiology. *American Journal of Physiology* 279: 743–55.

Smith, J. E. 1978. *Purpose and Thought: The Meaning of American Pragmatism.* New Haven, Conn.: Yale University Press.

Spector, A. C. 2000. Linking gustatory neurobiology to behavior in vertebrates. *Neuroscience and Biobehavioral Reviews* 24:391–416.

Spinoza, B. 1668/1955. *On the Improvement of the Understanding.* New York: Dover Press.

Starling, E. H. 1923. *The Wisdom of the Body.* London: H. K. Lewis.

Stellar, E. 1954. The physiology of motivation. *Psychological Review* 61:5–22.

———. 1989. Curt P. Richter. In *American Philosophical Society Biographical Memoirs,* 297–93. Philadelphia: American Philosophical Society.

Stephan, F. K., and I. Zucker. 1972. Circadian rhythms in behavior and locomotor activity of rats are eliminated by hypothalamic lesions. *Proceedings of the National Academy of Sciences USA* 69:1583–86.

Stewart, C. S. 1898. Variations in daily activity produced by alcohol and by changes in barometric pressure and diet with a description of recording methods. *American Journal of Physiology* 1:40–56.

Stricker, E. M. 1990. *Handbook of Behavioral Neurobiology*, vol. 10, *Neurobiology of Food and Fluid Intake*. New York: Plenum Press.

Thiels, E., J. G. Verbalis, and E. M. Stricker. 1990. Sodium appetite in lactating rats. *Behavioral Neuroscience* 104:742–50.

Thorpe, W. H. 1948. The modern concept of instinctive behaviour. *Bulletin of Animal Behaviour* 7:12–48.

Tinbergen, N. 1951/1969. *The Study of Instinct*. New York: Oxford University Press.

Titchener, E. B. 1929/1972. *Systemic Psychology*. Ithaca, N.Y.: Cornell University Press.

Todes, D. P. 2002. *Pavlov's Physiology Factory*. Baltimore: Johns Hopkins University Press.

Tolman, E. C. 1949. *Purposive Behavior in Animals and Men*. Berkeley: University of California Press.

Tordoff, M. G. 2001. Calcium: Taste, intake, and appetite. *Physiological Reviews* 81: 1567–97.

———. 2002. Obesity by choice: The powerful influence of nutrient availability on nutrient intake. *American Journal of Physiology* 282:R1536–39.

Von Frisch, K. 1956. Lernvermogen und erbgebundene Tradition Im Leben der Bienen. In *L'instinct dans le comportement des animaux et de l'homme*, edited by P. P. Grasse, chap. 10. Paris: Masson et Cie Editeurs.

Wada, T. 1922. An experimental study of hunger in its relation to activity. *Archives of Psychology*.

Watson, J. B. 1912. Instinctive activity in animals. *Harper's Magazine* 124:376–82.

———. 1919. *Psychology from the Standpoint of the Behaviorist*. Philadelphia: Lippincott.

———. 1924. *Behaviorism*. New York: W. W. Norton.

———. 1930/1961. Autobiography. In *A History of Psychology in Autobiography*. New York: Russell & Russell.

Wehr, T. A., D. E. Moul, G. Barbato, H. A. Giesen, J. A. Seidel, C. Barker, and C. Bender. 1993. Conservation of photoperiod-responsive mechanisms in humans. *American Journal of Physiology* 265:R846–57.

Weidman, N. M. 1999. *Constructing Scientific Psychology: Karl Lashley Mind-Brain Debates*. Cambridge: Cambridge University Press.

Weisinger, R. S., and S. C. Woods. 1971. Aldosterone-elicited sodium appetite. *Endocrinology* 89:538–44.

Wirth, J. B. 1989. Richter and Magendie. Talk given in celebration of Curt Richter at the Johns Hopkins University.

Wirth, J. B., and P. R. McHugh. 1983. Gastric distension and short term satiety in the rhesus monkey. *American Journal of Physiology* 245:174–80.

Wolf, G. 1964. Sodium appetite elicited by aldosterone. *Psychonomic Science* 1:211–12.

———. 1969. Innate mechanisms for regulation of sodium intake. In *Olfaction and Taste*, edited by C. Pfaffman, 548–53. New York: Rockefeller University Press.

Wolfe, E. L., A. C. Barger, and S. Benison. 2000. *Walter B. Cannon: Science and Society.* Cambridge: Harvard University Press.

Woodside, B., and L. Millelire. 1987. Self-selection of calcium during pregnancy and lactation in rats. *Physiology and Behavior* 39:391–97.

Yerkes, R. M. 1903. The associative processes of the green frog. *Psychological Review* 17:579–638.

———. 1913. The heredity of savageness and wildness in rats. *Journal of Animal Behavior* 2:286–96.

———. 1921. The relations of psychology to medicine. *Science* 53:106–11.

———. 1930. Autobiography of Robert Mearns Yerkes. In *History of Psychology in Autobiography*, edited by C. Murchison. Worcester, Mass.: Clark University Press.

Young, P. T. 1948. Appetite, palatability and feeding habit: A critical review. *Psychological Bulletin* 45:289–320.

THE WORKS OF CURT RICHTER

This bibliography is derived from Elliot Blass's edited book *The Psychobiology of Curt Richter,* a wonderful collection of Richter's work. Blass was a professor of psychobiology in the Department of Psychology at the Johns Hopkins University, and he went to great pains to enlist Richter's advice and then to capture the essential papers of Richter's work. Richter's wife, Leslie Richter, covered the costs of the edited book, a fact of which Richter was unaware (E. Blass, pers. comm., July 2002).

The Blass book includes Richter's publications through 1976, when it was published. To these I have added the papers that have come out subsequently.

Anderson, W. A., and C. P. Richter. 1946. Toxicity of alpha-naphthyl thiourea for chickens and pigs. *Veterinary Medicine* 41:302–3.

Bagley, C. J., and C. P. Richter. 1924. Electrically excitable region of the forebrain of the alligator. *Archives of Neurology and Psychiatry* 2:257–63.

Barelare, B., Jr., L. E. Holt Jr., and C. P. Richter. 1938. Influence of vitamin deficiencies on appetite for particular foodstuffs. *American Journal of Physiology* 123:7–8.

Barelare, B., Jr., and C. P. Richter. 1938. Increased sodium chloride appetite in pregnant rats. *American Journal of Physiology* 121:185–88.

Bordley, J. E., W. G. Hardy, and C. P. Richter. 1948. Audiometry with the use of galvanic skin resistance response. *Bulletin of the Johns Hopkins Hospital* 82:569–77.

Bruesch, S. R., and C. P. Richter. 1946. Cutaneous distribution of peripheral nerves in rhesus monkeys as determined by the electric skin resistance method. *Bulletin of the Johns Hopkins Hospital* 78:235–48.

Buchman, E. F., and C. P. Richter. 1933. Abolition of bulbocapnine catatonia by cocaine. *Archives of Neurology and Psychiatry* 29:499–503.

Carter, E. P., C. P. Richter, and C. H. Greene. 1919. A graphic application of the principle of the equilateral triangle for determining the direction of the electrical axis of the heart in the human electrocardiogram. *Bulletin of the Johns Hopkins Hospital* 30: 162–67.

Dieke, S. H., G. S. Allen, and C. P. Richter. 1947. The acute toxicity of thioureas and related compounds to wild and domestic Norway rats. *Journal of Pharmacology and Experimental Therapeutics* 90:260–70.

Dieke, S. H., and C. P. Richter. 1945. Acute toxicity of thiourea to rats in relation to age, diet, strain, and species variation. *Journal of Pharmacology and Experimental Therapeutics* 83:195–202.

———. 1946a. Age and species variation in the acute toxicity of alpha-naphthyl thiourea. *Proceedings of the Society for Experimental Biology and Medicine* 62:22–25.

———. 1946b. Comparative assays of rodenticides on wild Norway rats. I. Toxicity. *Public Health Reports* 61:672–79.

Fish, H. S., P. D. Malone, and C. P. Richter. 1944. The anatomy of the tongue of the domestic Norway rat. I. The skin of the tongue: The various papillae; their number and distribution. *Anatomical Record* 89:429–40.

Fish, H. S., and C. P. Richter. 1946. Comparative numbers of fungiform and foliate papillae on tongues of domestic and wild Norway rats. *Proceedings of the Society for Experimental Biology and Medicine* 63:352–55.

Fries, J. F., and C. P. Richter. 1964. Lung cancer: Detection by use of electrical skin resistance method. *Archives of Internal Medicine* 113:624–34.

Gillespie, R. D., C. P. Richter, and G. Wang. 1926. The oculo-cardiac reflex: its clinical significance. *Journal of Mental Science* 72:321–30.

King, A. B., and C. P. Richter. 1949. Spinal subdural abscess due to a congenital dermal sinus and accompanying changes in the autonomic nervous system. *Bulletin of the Johns Hopkins Hospital* 85:431–39.

Kline, A. H., J. B. Sidbury Jr., and C. P. Richter. 1959. The occurrence of ectodermal dysplasia and corneal dysplasia in one family. *Journal of Pediatrics* 55:355–66.

Kline, A. H., J. B. Sidbury Jr., C. P. Richter, and J. Billingsly. 1959. Mode of transmission of familial ectodermal dysplasia. *American Pediatric Society* 55:355–66.

Langworthy, O. R., and C. P. Richter. 1930. The influence of efferent cerebral pathways upon the sympathetic nervous system. *Brain* 53:178–93.

———. 1933. The cerebral motor cortex of the porcupine. *Journal of Psychology and Neurology* 45:138–42.

———. 1938. A physiological study of cerebral motor cortex and decerebrate rigidity in the beaver. *Journal of Mammalogy* 19:70–77.

———. 1939. Increased spontaneous activity produced by frontal lobe lesions in cats. *American Journal of Physiology* 126:158–61.

Levine, M., and C. P. Richter. 1935. Periodic attacks of gastric pain accompanied with marked changes in the electrical resistance of the skin. *Archives of Neurology and Psychiatry* 33:1078–80.

Mirick, G. S., C. P. Richter, I. G. Schaub, R. Franklin, R. MacCleary, G. Schipper, and J. Spitznagel. 1950. An epizootic due to pneumococcus type II in laboratory rats. *American Journal of Hygiene* 52:48–54.

Mosier, H. D., Jr., and C. P. Richter. 1958. Response of the glomerulosa layer of the adrenal gland of wild and domesticated Norway rats to low and high salt diets. *Endocrinology* 62:268–77.

Mosier, H. D., Jr., and C. P. Richter. 1967. Histologic and physiologic comparisons of the thyroid glands of the wild and domesticated Norway rat. *Anatomical Record* 158:263–74.

Park, E. A., and C. P. Richter. 1953. Transverse lines in bones: The mechanism of their development. *Bulletin of the Johns Hopkins Hospital* 93:234–48.

Paterson, A. S., and C. P. Richter. 1933. Action of scopolamine and carbon dioxide on catalepsy produced by bulbocapnine. *Archives of Neurology and Psychiatry* 29:231–40.

Pfaffmann, C., P. T. Young, V. G. Dethier, C. P. Richter, and E. Stellar. 1954. Preparation of solution for research in chemoreception and food acceptance. *Journal of Comparative Physiology and Psychology* 47:93–96.

Rice, K. K., and C. P. Richter. 1943. Increased sodium chloride and water intake of normal rats treated with desoxycorticosterone acetate. *Endocrinology* 33:106–15.

Richter, C. P. 1921. The behavior of the rat: a study of general and specific activities. Ph.D. diss., Johns Hopkins Univ.

———. 1922. A behavioristic study of the activity of the rat. *Comparative Psychology Monographs* 1:1–55.

———. 1924a. Action currents from the stomach. *American Journal of Physiology* 67:612–33.

———. 1924b. The sweat glands studied by the electrical resistance method. *American Journal of Physiology* 68:147.

———. 1925. Some observations on the self-stimulation habits of young wild animals. *Archives of Neurology and Psychiatry* 13:724–28.

———. 1926a. New methods of obtaining electromyogram and electrocardiogram from the intact body. *JAMA* 87:1300.

———. 1926b. The significance of changes in the electrical resistance of the body during sleep. *Proceedings of the National Academy of Sciences* 12:214–22.

———. 1926c. A study of the effect of moderate doses of alcohol on the growth and behavior of the rat. *Journal of Experimental Zoology* 44:397–418.

———. 1927a. Animal behavior and internal drives. *Quarterly Review of Biology* 2:307–43.

———. 1927b. On the interpretation of the electromyogram from voluntary and reflex contractions. *Quarterly Journal of Experimental Physiology* 18:55–77.

———. 1927c. A study of the electrical skin resistance and the psychogalvanic reflex in a case of unilateral sweating. *Brain* 50:216–23.

———. 1928a. The dependence of the electromyogram from voluntary contractions on the anterior horn cells. *American Journal of Physiology* 85:403–23.

———. 1928b. The electrical skin resistance. *Archives of Neurology and Psychiatry* 19:488–508.

————. 1929a. The galvanic skin-reflex in spinal animals. *Proceedings and Papers of the Ninth International Congress on Psychology,* 357–58.

————. 1929b. Nervous control of the electrical resistance of the skin. *Bulletin of the Johns Hopkins Hospital* 45:56–74.

————. 1929c. Pathologic sleep and similar conditions. *Archives of Neurology and Psychiatry* 21:363–75.

————. 1929d. Physiological factors involved in the electrical resistance of the skin. *American Journal of Physiology* 88:596–615.

————. 1929e. Thirst: A function of body-surface. *Proceedings and Papers of the Ninth International Congress on Psychology,* 358–59.

————. 1930a. Biological approach to manic depressive insanity. *Proceedings of the Association for Research in Nervous and Mental Disease* 11:611–25.

————. 1930b. Experimental diabetes insipidus. *Brain* 53:76–85.

————. 1930c. Galvanic skin reflex from animals with complete transection of the spinal cord. *American Journal of Physiology* 93:468–72.

————. 1930d. High electrical resistance of the skin of new-born infants and its significance. *American Journal of Diseases of Children* 40:18–26.

————. 1931a. The grasping reflex in the new-born monkey. *Archives of Neurology and Psychiatry* 26:784–90.

————. 1931b. Sleep produced by hypnotics studied by the electrical skin resistance method. *Journal of Pharmacology and Experimental Therapeutics* 42:471–86.

————. 1932. Biological foundation of personality differences. *American Journal of Orthopsychiatry* 2:345–54.

————. 1933a. Cyclical phenomena produced in rats by section of the pituitary stalk and their possible relation to pseudo-pregnancy. *American Journal of Physiology* 106:80–90.

————. 1933b. The effect of early gonadectomy on the gross body activity of rats. *Endocrinology* 17:445–50.

————. 1933c. The role played by the thyroid gland in the production of gross body activity. *Endocrinology* 17:73–87.

————. 1934a. Cyclic manifestations in the sleep curves of psychotic patients. *Archives of Neurology and Psychiatry* 31:149–51.

————. 1934b. Experimental diabetes insipidus: its relation to the anterior and posterior lobes of the hypophysis. *American Journal of Physiology* 110:439–47.

————. 1934c. The grasp reflex of the new-born infant. *American Journal of Diseases of Children* 48:327–32.

————. 1934d. Pregnancy urine given by mouth to gonadectomized rats: its effect on spontaneous activity and on the reproductive tract. *American Journal of Physiology* 110:499–512.

————. 1935. The primacy of polyuria in diabetes insipidus. *American Journal of Physiology* 112:481–87.

———. 1936a. Increased salt appetite in adrenalectomized rats. *American Journal of Physiology* 115:155–61.

———. 1936b. The pituitary gland in relation to water exchange. *Proceedings of the Association for Research in Nervous and Mental Disease* 17:392–409.

———. 1936c. The spontaneous activity of adrenalectomized rats treated with replacement and other therapy. *Endocrinology* 20:657–66.

———. 1937. Hypophyseal control of behavior. *Cold Spring Harbor Symposia on Quantitative Biology* 5:258–68.

———. 1938a. Animal cages. *American Journal of Physiology* 123:170.

———. 1938b. Factors determining voluntary ingestion of water in normals and in individuals with maximum diabetes insipidus. *American Journal of Physiology* 122:668–75.

———. 1938c. The integration of the grasp reflex. *Transactions of the American Neurological Association*, 64th meeting, 128.

———. 1938d. Two-day cycles of alternating good and bad behavior in psychotic patients. *Archives of Neurology and Psychiatry* 39:587–98.

———. 1938e. The work of the psychobiology laboratory. In *Contributions Dedicated to Dr. Adolf Meyer*, edited by S. Katzenelbogen, 81–85. Baltimore: Johns Hopkins University.

———. 1939a. Salt taste thresholds of normal and adrenalectomized rats. *Endocrinology* 24:367–71.

———. 1939b. Transmission of taste sensation in animals. *Transactions of the American Neurological Association*, 65th meeting, 49–50.

———. 1941a. Alcohol as a food. *Quarterly Journal of Studies on Alcohol* 1:650–62.

———. 1941b. Behavior and endocrine regulators of the internal environment. *Endocrinology* 28:193–95.

———. 1941c. Biology of drives. *Psychosomatic Medicine* 3:105–10.

———. 1941d. Changes produced by sympathectomy in the electrical resistance of the skin. *Transactions of the American Neurological Association*, 67th meeting, 15–17.

———. 1941e. Decreased carbohydrate appetite of adrenalectomized rats. *Proceedings of the Society for Experimental Biology and Medicine* 48:577–79.

———. 1941f. The internal environment and behavior. Internal secretions. *American Journal of Psychiatry* 97:878–93.

———. 1941g. The nutritional value of some common carbohydrates, fats and proteins studied in rats by the single food choice method. *American Journal of Physiology* 133:29–42.

———. 1941h. Sodium chloride and dextrose appetite of untreated and treated adrenalectomized rats. *Endocrinology* 29:115–25.

———. 1942a. Increased dextrose appetite of normal rats treated with insulin. *American Journal of Physiology* 135:781–87.

———. 1942b. Physiological psychology. *Annual Review of Physiology* 4:561–74.

———. 1942–43. Total self regulatory functions in animals and human beings. *Harvey Lectures Series* 38:63–103.

———. 1943. The self-selection of diets. In *Essays in Biology: In Honor of Herbert M. Evans*, edited by S. T. Farquhar, C. D. Leak, W. R. Lyons, and M. E. Simpson. Berkeley: University of California Press.

———. 1945a. A comparison of the nutritive values of dextrose and of corn syrups and of the effects produced on their utilization by thiamine. *American Journal of Physiology* 145:107–14.

———. 1945b. The development and use of alpha-naphthyl thiourea (ANTU) as a rat poison. *JAMA* 129:927–31.

———. 1945c. Incidence of rat bites and rat bite fever in Baltimore. *JAMA* 128:324–26.

———. 1945d. Nutritive value of dextrose maltose determined by the single-food choice method. *Proceedings of the Society for Experimental Biology and Medicine* 59: 260–63.

———. 1946a. Biological factors involved in poisoning rats with alpha-naphthyl thiourea (ANTU). *Proceedings of the Society for Experimental Biology and Medicine* 63: 364–72.

———. 1946b. Instructions for using the cutaneous resistance recorder, or "dermometer," on peripheral nerve injuries, sympathectomies, and paravertebral blocks. *Journal of Neurosurgery* 3:181–91.

———. 1947a. Biology of drives. *Journal of Comparative Physiology and Psychology* 40: 129–34.

———. 1947b. Cutaneous areas denervated by upper thoracic and stellate ganglionectomies determined by the electrical skin resistance method. *Journal of Neurosurgery* 4:221–32.

———. 1948a. Effect of galactose on the utilization of fat. *Science* 108:449–50.

———. 1948b. Nutritive value of fructose for rats and effects produced on its utilization by thiamine. *American Journal of Physiology* 154:499–505.

———. 1948c. Physiology and endocrinology of the toxic thioureas. *Recent Progress in Hormone Research* 11:255–76.

———. 1949a. Domestication of the Norway rat and its implications for the problem of stress. *Proceedings of the Association for Research in Nervous and Mental Disease* 29: 19–47.

———. 1949b. The use of the wild Norway rat for psychiatric research. *Journal of Nervous and Mental Disease* 110:379–86.

———. 1950a. An ideal preparation for the dissection of spinal, peripheral and autonomic nerves of the rat. *Science* 112:20–21.

———. 1950b. Psychotic behavior produced in wild Norway and Alexandrine rats apparently by the fear of poisoning. In *International Symposium on Feelings and Emotions*, edited by M. L. Reymert, 189–202. New York: McGraw Hill.

———. 1950c. Taste and solubility of toxic compounds in poisoning of rats and man. *Journal of Comparative Physiology and Psychology* 43:358–74.

———. 1951. The effects of domestication on the steroids of animals and man. *Symposium on Steroids and Behavior*, Ciba Foundation, London, England.

———. 1952a. Domestication of the Norway rat and its implication for the study of genetics in man. *American Journal of Human Genetics* 4:273–85.

———. 1952b. The physiology and cytology of pulmonary edema and pleural effusion produced in rats by alpha-naphthyl thiourea (ANTU). *Journal of Thoracic Surgery* 23:66–91.

———. 1952c. *Stress and Structural Change.* Seventh annual Menas S. Gregory Lecture at New York University–Bellevue Medical Center.

———. 1953a. Alcohol, beer and wine as foods. *Quarterly Journal of Studies on Alcohol* 14:525–39.

———. 1953b. *Behavioral Regulation of Homeostasis.* Symposium on Stress. Army Medical Service Graduate School, Walter Reed Army Medical Center, Washington, D.C.

———. 1953c. Behavior cycles in man and animals. *National Academy of Sciences.*

———. 1953d. Experimentally produced behavior reactions to food poisoning in wild and domesticated rats. *Annals of the New York Academy of Sciences* 56:225–39.

———. 1953e. Experimental production of cycles of behaviour and physiology in animals. *Acta Medica Scandinavica, Supplementum* 307:36.

———. 1953f. Free research versus design research. *Science* 118:91–93.

———. 1954a. Behavioral regulators of carbohydrate homeostasis. *Acta Neurovegetativa* 9:247–69.

———. 1954b. The effects of domestication and selection on the behavior of the Norway rat. *Journal of the National Cancer Institute* 15:727–38.

———. 1955a. Behavior and metabolic cycles in animals and man. *Proceedings of the 45th Annual Meeting of the American Psychopathological Association Experimental Psychopathology*, edited by Hoch and Zublin, 34–54. New York: Grune and Stratton.

———. 1955b. Nutritional factors. Report of the *17th Ross Pediatric Research Conference on Growth and Development of Dental and Skeletal Tissues*, Boston, Mass., 22–30.

———. 1955c. Self-regulatory functions during gestation and lactation. *Gestation-Transactions of the Second Conference*, Princeton, N.J., 11–93.

———. 1956a. Loss of appetite for alcohol and alcoholic beverages produced in rats by treatment with thyroid preparations. *Endocrinology* 59:472–78.

———. 1956b. Ovulation cycles and stress. *Transactions of the 3rd Conference on Gestation*, Princeton, N.J., edited by C. A. Villee, 53–70.

———. 1956c. Production and control of alcoholic cravings in rats. *Third Conference in Neuropharmacology*, Princeton, N.J., edited by H. A. Abramson, 39–146. New York: The Josiah Macy Jr. Foundation.

———. 1956d. Salt appetite of mammals: its dependence on instinct and metabolism. In *L'Instinct dans le comportement des animaux et de l'homme*, edited by P. P. Grasse, 577–632. Paris: Masson et Cie Editeurs.

———. 1957a. Decreased appetite for alcohol and alcoholic beverages produced in rats by thyroid treatment. *Symposium on hormones, brain function and behavior. Proceedings of the Conference on Neuroendocrinology*, edited by H. Hoagland, 217–20. New York: Academic Press.

———. 1957b. Hormones and rhythms in man and animals. *Recent Progress in Hormone Research* 13:105–59, edited by Gregory Pincus. New York: Academic Press.

———. 1957c. Hunger and appetite. *American Journal of Clinical Nutrition* 5:141.

———. 1957d. Loss of appetite for alcohol and alcoholic beverages produced in rats by treatment with thyroid preparation. *Symposium on Alcoholism-Basic Aspects and Treatment*, Atlanta, Ga., edited by H. E. Himwich. American Association for the Advancement of Science, publ. no. 47.

———. 1957e. Permanent damage done to rats by prolonged feeding of several common therapeutic drugs and hormones. *Proceedings of the National Academy of Sciences* 126:1234.

———. 1957f. Phenomenon of sudden death in animals and man. *Psychosomatic Medicine* 19:191–98.

———. 1958a. Abnormal but regular cycles in behavior and metabolism in rats and catatonic-schizophrenics. In *Psychoendocrinology*, edited by M. Reiss, 168–81. New York: Grune and Stratton.

———. 1958b. Diurnal cycles of man and animals. *Science* 128:1147–48.

———. 1958c. Neurological basis of responses to stress. *A Ciba Foundation Symposium on the Neurological Basis of Behaviour*, in commemoration of Sir Charles Sherrington, edited by G. E. W. Wolstenholme and Cecilia M. O'Connor, 204–17. London: J. and A. Churchill.

———. 1958d. On the phenomenon of sudden death in animals and man. In *Psychopathology: A Source Book*, edited by C. F. Reed, I. E. Alexander, and S. S. Tomkins, 112–25. Cambridge: Harvard University Press.

———. 1958e. The phenomenon of unexplained sudden death in animals and man. (Article read at the 25th anniversary of the Pavlovian Laboratory, Phipps Psychiatric Clinic, Johns Hopkins Hospital.) In *Physiological Bases of Psychiatry*, compiled and edited by W. H. Gantt, 302–13.

———. 1959a. Abnormal but regular cycles in behavior and metabolism in rats and catatonic-schizophrenics. *Second International Congress of Psychiatry, Psychoendocrine Symposium with Special Reference to Schizophrenia*, Zurich, Switzerland, 1957. 4:326–27.

———. 1959b. *Biological Clocks in Medicine and Psychiatry*. Thomas William Salmon Lectures at the New York Academy of Medicine.

———. 1959c. Lasting after-effects produced in rats by several commonly used drugs and hormones. *Proceedings of the National Academy of Sciences* 45:1080–95.

———. 1959d. Rats, man and the welfare state. *American Psychologist* 14:18–28.

———. 1960. Biological clocks in medicine and psychiatry: Shock-phase hypothesis. *Proceedings of the National Academy of Sciences* 46:1506–30.

———. 1961a. Biological clocks. Presented at the annual meeting of the American Philosophical Society, Philadelphia, Pa.

———. 1961b. Biological clocks in infants and children. Presented at the annual meeting of the American Pediatrics Society.

———. 1964a. Behavioral and physiological changes produced in rats by removal of the superior colliculi of the brain. Presented at the National Academy of Sciences autumn meeting, University of Wisconsin, Madison, October 12–14, 1964. *Science* 146:429.

———. 1964b. Biological clocks and the endocrine glands. *Proceedings of the Second International Congress of Endocrinology*, London, England, 119–23.

———. 1965. *Biological Clocks in Medicine and Psychiatry*. Springfield, Ill.: Charles C. Thomas.

———. 1966. A hitherto unrecognized difference between man and other primates. *Science* 154:427.

———. 1967a. Biological clocks. *Ciba Foundation Meeting*, in honor of Professor Bernhard Zondek, London, England, July 27, 1966, edited by G. E. W. Wolstenholme. London: J. & A. Churchill.

———. 1967b. Psychopathology of periodic behavior in animals and man. *Comparative Psychopathology*. American Psychopathological Association/New York: Grune & Stratton, 205–27.

———. 1967c. Sleep and activity: Their relation to the 24-hour clock. *Proceedings of the Association for Research on Nervous and Mental Disease* 45:8–29.

———. 1968a. Clock mechanism esotropia in children-alternate-day squint. *Johns Hopkins Medical Journal* 122:218–23.

———. 1968b. Experiences of a reluctant rat-catcher: The common Norway rat—friend or enemy? *Proceedings of the Philosophical Society* 112:403–15.

———. 1968c. Inborn nature of the rat's 24-hour clock. *Proceedings of the National Academy of Sciences* 61:1153–54.

———. 1968d. Inherent twenty-four hour and lunar clocks of a primate—the squirrel monkey. *Comparative Behavioral Biology* part A, 1:305–32.

———. 1968e. Periodic phenomena in man and animals: their relation to neuroendocrine mechanisms (a monthly or nearly monthly cycle). In *Endocrinology and Human Behaviour*, edited by R. P. Michael. London: Oxford University Press.

———. 1970a. Blood-clock barrier: Its penetration by heavy water. *Proceedings of the National Academy of Sciences* 66:244.

————. 1970b. Dependence of successful mating in rats on functioning of the 24-hour clocks of the male and female. *Comparative Behavioral Biology* part A, 5: no. 1.

————. 1970d. Yogurt induced cataracts: Comments on their significance to man. *JAMA* 214:1878–79.

————. 1971. Inborn nature of the rat's 24-hour clock. *Journal of Comparative Physiology and Psychology* 75:1–4.

————. 1972. Measurement of the electrical skin resistance in the evaluation of patients with neck and upper extremity pain. *Journal of Bone and Joint Surgery* 54:1796.

————. 1974. Part played by taste in self-selection of diets as determined by six common sugars. *Conference on the Development of Sweet Preference*, sponsored by the National Institute of Dental Research, Bethesda, Md.

————. 1975a. Astronomical references in biological rhythms. *International Society for the Study of Time, Second World Conference*, Lake Yamanaka, Japan. New York: Springer-Verlag.

————. 1975b. Deep hypothermia and its effect on the 24-hour clock of rats and hamsters. *Johns Hopkins Medical Journal* 136:1–10.

————. 1976a. Artifactual 7 day cycles in spontaneous activity in wild rodents and squirrel monkeys. *Journal of Comparative and Physiological Psychology* 90:572–82.

————. 1976b. Optic nerve sectioning in rats. *Brain Research Bulletin* 1:493–94.

————. 1977a. Discovery of fire by man: its effects on his 24 hour clock and intellectual and cultural evolution. *Johns Hopkins Medical Journal* 141:47–61.

————. 1977b. Heavy water as a tool for study of the forces that control length of period of the 24 hour clock of the hamster. *Proceedings of the National Academy of Sciences USA* 74:1295–99.

————. 1977c. Mysterious form of referred sensation in man. *Proceedings of the National Academy of Sciences USA* 74:4702–5.

————. 1977d. Permanent series of prolonged pseudopregnancy periods in hysterectomized rats. *Physiology and Behavior* 18:245–53.

————. 1978a. Dark active rat transformed into light active rat by destruction of 24-hour clock: function of 24-hour clock and synchronizers. *Proceedings of the National Academy of Sciences USA* 75:6276–80.

————. 1978b. Evidence for existence of a yearly clock in surgically and self blinded chipmunks. *Proceedings of the National Academy of Sciences USA* 75:3517–21.

————. 1980. Growth hormone 3.6-h pulsatile secretion and feeding times have similar periods in rats. *American Journal of Physiology* 239:E1–2.

————. 1983. Possible origin of a 90 min. cortisol secretion cycle in rats, guinea pigs and monkeys. *American Journal of Physiology* 244:R514–15.

————. 1985. It's a long way to Tipperary, the land of my genes. In *Leaders in the Study of Animal Behavior: Autobiographical Perspectives*, edited by D. A. Dewsbury, 357–85. Lewisburg, Pa.: Bucknell University Press.

Richter, C. P., and B. Barelare Jr. 1938. Nutritional requirements of pregnant and lactating rats studied by the self-selection method. *Endocrinology* 23:15–24.

———. 1939a. Further observations on the carbohydrate, fat, and protein appetite of vitamin B deficient rats. *American Journal of Physiology* 127:199–210.

———. 1939b. Persistence of 4- to 5-day activity cycles in vitamin A deficient rats with constant cornification of the vaginal epithelium. *Endocrinology* 24:3764–66.

Richter, C. P., and L. H. Bartemeier. 1926. Decerebrate rigidity of the sloth. *Brain* 49: 207–27.

Richter, C. P., and J. A. Benjamin Jr. 1934a. Ligation of the common bile duct in the rat. *Archives of Pathology* 18:817–26.

———. 1934b. The third ventricle: Conformation of the floor and its relation to the meninges. *Archives of Neurology and Psychiatry* 31:1026–37.

Richter, C. P., and J. R. Birmingham. 1941. Calcium appetite of parathyroidectomized rats used to bioassay substances which affect blood calcium. *Endocrinology* 29: 655–66.

———. 1942. Decreased fat appetite produced in rats by ligation of the common bile duct. *American Journal of Physiology* 138:71–77.

Richter, C. P., and M. E. Brailey. 1929. Water-intake and its relation to the surface area of the body. *Proceedings of the National Academy of Sciences* 15:571–78.

Richter, C. P., and K. H. Campbell. 1940a. Alcohol taste thresholds and concentrations of solution preferred by rats. *Science* 91:507–8.

———. 1940b. Sucrose taste thresholds of rats and humans. *American Journal of Physiology* 128:291–97.

———. 1940c. Taste thresholds and taste preferences of rats for five common sugars. *Journal of Nutrition* 20:31–46.

Richter, C. P., and K. H. Clisby. 1941a. Graying of hair produced by ingestion of phenylthiocarbamide. *Proceedings of the Society for Experimental Biology and Medicine* 48:684–87.

———. 1941b. Phenylthiocarbamide taste thresholds of rats and human beings. *American Journal of Physiology* 134:157–64.

———. 1942. Toxic effects of the bitter-tasting phenylthiocarbamide. *Archives of Pathology* 33:46–57.

Richter, C. P., and J. R. Duke. 1970. Cataracts produced in rats by yogurt. *Science* 168: 1372–74.

Richter, C. P., and J. F. Eckert. 1935. Further evidence for the primacy of polyuria in diabetes insipidus. *American Journal of Physiology* 113:578–81.

———. 1936. Behavior changes produced in the rat by hypophysectomy. *Proceedings of the Association for Research in Nervous and Mental Disease.* 17:561–71.

———. 1937a. The effect of hypophyseal injection and implants on the activity of hypophysectomized rats. *Endocrinology* 21:481–88.

————. 1937b. Increased calcium appetite of parathyroidectomized rats. *Endocrinology* 21:50–54.

————. 1938. Mineral metabolism of adrenalectomized rats studied by the appetite method. *Endocrinology* 22:214–24.

————. 1939. Mineral appetite of parathyroidectomized rats. *American Journal of the Medical Sciences* 198:9–16.

Richter, C. P., and J. T. Emlen Jr. 1945. A modified rabbit box trap for use in catching live wild rats for laboratory and field studies. *Public Health Reports* 60:1303–8.

————. 1946. Instructions for using ANTU as a poison for the common Norway rat. *Public Health Reports* 61:602–7.

Richter, C. P., and F. R. Ford. 1928. Electromyographic studies in different types of neuromuscular disturbances. *Archives of Neurology and Psychiatry* 19:660–76.

Richter, C. P., and C. E. Hall. 1947. Comparison of intestinal lengths and Peyer's patches in wild and domestic Norway and in wild Alexandrine rats. *Proceedings of the Society for Experimental Biology and Medicine* 66:561–66.

Richter, C. P., and C. G. Hartman. 1934. The effect of injection of amniotin on the spontaneous activity of gonadectomized rats. *American Journal of Physiology* 108:136–43.

Richter, C. P., and C. D. Hawkes. 1939. Increased spontaneous activity and food intake produced in rats by removal of the frontal poles of the brain. *Journal of Neurology and Psychiatry* 2:231–42.

————. 1941. The dependence of the carbohydrate, fat and protein appetite of rats on the various components of the vitamin B complex. *American Journal of Physiology* 131:639–49.

Richter, C. P., and S. Helfrick. 1943. Decreased phosphorous appetite of parathyroidectomized rats. *Endocrinology* 33:349–52.

Richter, C. P., and M. Hines. 1932a. Experimental production of the grasp reflex in adult monkeys by lesions of the frontal lobes. *American Journal of Physiology* 101:87–99.

————. 1932b. The production of the "grasp reflex" in adult macaques by experimental frontal lobe lesions. *Proceedings of the Association for Research in Nervous and Mental Disease* 13:211–24.

————. 1935. Increased activity produced by brain lesions in monkeys. *Second International Neurological Congress.*

————. 1937. Increased general activity produced by pre-frontal and striatal lesions in monkeys. *Transactions of the American Neurological Association*, 63rd meeting, 107–9.

————. 1938. Increased spontaneous activity produced in monkeys by brain lesions. *Brain* 61:1–16.

Richter, C. P., L. E. Holt Jr., and B. Barelare Jr. 1937a. The effect of self-selection of diet—food (protein, carbohydrates, and fats), minerals and vitamins—on growth, activity, and reproduction in rats. *American Journal of Physiology* 119:388–89.

———. 1937b. Vitamin B1 craving in rats. *Science* 86:354–55.

———. 1938. Nutritional requirements for normal growth and reproduction in rats studied by the self-selection method. *American Journal of Physiology* 122:734–44.

Richter, C. P., L. E. Holt Jr., B. Barelare Jr., and C. D. Hawkes. 1939. Changes in fat, carbohydrate, and protein appetite in vitamin B deficiency. *American Journal of Physiology* 124:596–602.

Richter, C. P., W. Honeyman, and H. Hunter. 1940. Behavior and mood cycles apparently related to parathyroid deficiency. *Journal of Neurology and Psychiatry* 3:19–25.

Richter, C. P., G. E. S. Jones, and L. Biswanger. 1959. Periodic phenomena and the thyroid. I. Abnormal but regular cycles in behavior and metabolism produced in rats by partial radiothyroidectomy. *Archives of Neurology and Psychiatry* 81:233–55.

Richter, C. P., G. E. S. Jones, and J. W. Woods. 1953. Behavior cycles produced in rats by thyroidectomy, injection of I^{131}, or by feeding sulfamerazine. *Endocrinology.*

Richter, C. P., and D. T. Katz. 1943. Peripheral nerve injuries determined by the electrical skin resistance method. I. Ulnar nerve. *JAMA* 122:648–51.

Richter, C. P., and O. R. Langworthy. 1933. The quill mechanism of the porcupine. *Journal of Psychology and Neurology* 45:143–53.

Richter, C. P., O. R. Langworthy, and E. A. Park. 1967. An ideal preparation of animals (on single-food-choice diet) for dissection of nerves and glands and for bone growth studies. *Proceedings of the National Academy of Sciences* 57:265–72.

Richter, C. P., and M. Levine. 1937. Sympathectomy in man. *Archives of Neurology and Psychiatry* 38:756–60.

Richter, C. P., and A. MacLean. 1939. Salt taste thresholds of humans. *American Journal of Physiology* 126:1–6.

Richter, C. P., and P. D. Malone. 1945. Peripheral nerve lesion charts. *Journal of Neurosurgery* 2:550–52.

Richter, C. P., and H. D. Mosier Jr. 1954. Maximum sodium chloride intake and thirst in domesticated and wild Norway rats. *American Journal of Physiology* 176:213–22.

Richter, C. P., and F. J. Otenasek. 1946. Thoracolumbar sympathectomies examined with the electrical skin resistance method. *Journal of Neurosurgery* 3:120–34.

Richter, C. P., and A. S. Paterson. 1931. Bulbocapnine catalepsy and the grasp reflex. *Journal of Pharmacology and Experimental Therapeutics* 43:677–91.

———. 1932. On the pharmacology of the grasp reflex. *Brain* 55:391–96.

Richter, C. P., and K. K. Rice. 1942. The effect of thiamine hydrochloride on the energy value of dextrose studied in rats by the single food choice method. *American Journal of Physiology* 137:573–81.

———. 1943a. Depressive effects produced on appetite and activity of rats by an exclusive diet of yellow or white corn and their correction by cod liver oil. *American Journal of Physiology* 139:147–54.

————. 1943b. Effects produced by vitamin D on energy, appetite, and oestrous cycles of rats kept on an exclusive diet of yellow corn. *American Journal of Physiology* 139: 693–99.

————. 1944. Comparison of the nutritive value of dextrose and casein and of the effects produced by their utilization by thiamine. *American Journal of Physiology* 141: 346–53.

————. 1945a. A comparison of the nutritive value of dextrose and sucrose and of the effects produced on their utilization by thiamine hydrochloride. *American Journal of Physiology* 143:336–43.

————. 1945b. Self-selection studies on coprophagy as a source of vitamin B complex. *American Journal of Physiology* 143:344–54.

————. 1954. Comparison of the effects produced by fasting on gross bodily activity of wild and domesticated Norway rats. *American Journal of Physiology* 179:305–8.

————. 1956. Experimental production in rats of abnormal cycles in behavior and metabolism. *Journal of Nervous and Mental Disease* 124:393–95.

Richter, C. P., P. V. Rogers, and C. E. Hall. 1950. Failure of salt replacement therapy in adrenalectomized recently captured wild Norway rats. *Endocrinology* 46:233–42.

Richter, C. P., and E. C. H. Schmidt Jr. 1939. Behavior and anatomical changes reproduced in rats by pancreatectomy. *Endocrinology* 25:698–706.

————. 1941. Increased fat and decreased carbohydrate appetite of pancreatectomized rats. *Endocrinology* 28:179–92.

Richter, C. P., E. C. H. Schmidt Jr., and P. D. Malone. 1945. Further observations on the self-regulatory dietary selections of rats made diabetic by pancreatectomy. *Bulletin of the Johns Hopkins Hospital* 76:192–219.

Richter, C. P., and M. B. Shaw. 1930. Complete transections of the spinal cord at different levels. *Archives of Neurology and Psychiatry* 24:1107–16.

Richter, C. P., and E. H. Uhlenhuth. 1954. Comparison of the effects of gonadectomy on spontaneous activity of wild and domesticated Norway rats. *Endocrinology* 54: 311–22.

Richter, C. P., and T. Wada. 1924. Method of measuring salivary secretions in human beings. *Journal of Laboratory and Clinical Medicine* 9:2–4.

Richter, C. P., and G. H. Wang. 1926. New apparatus for measuring the spontaneous motility of animals. *Journal of Laboratory and Clinical Medicine* 12:289–92.

Richter, C. P., and C. L. Warner. 1974. Comparison of Weigert stained sections with unfixed, unstained sections for study of myelin sheaths. *Proceedings of the National Academy of Sciences* 71:598–601.

Richter, C. P., and F. G. Whelan. 1943. Sweat gland responses to sympathetic stimulation studied by the galvanic skin reflex method. *Journal of Neurophysiology* 6:191–94.

————. 1949. Description of a skin galvanometer that gives a graphic record of activity in the sympathetic nervous system. *Journal of Neurosurgery* 6:279–84.

Richter, C. P., and G. B. Wislocki. 1928. Activity studies on castrated male and female rats with testicular grafts in correlation with histological studies of the grafts. *American Journal of Physiology* 86:651–60.

———. 1930. Anatomical and behavior changes produced in the rat by complete and partial extirpation of the pituitary gland. *American Journal of Physiology* 95:481–92.

Richter, C. P., and D. E. Wood. 1953. Hypophysectomy and domestication in the Norway rat. *Federal Proceedings* 12:378.

Richter, C. P., and B. G. Woodruff. 1941. Changes produced by sympathectomy in the electrical resistance of the skin. *Surgery* 10:957–70.

———. 1942. Facial patterns of electrical skin resistance: their relation to sleep, external temperature, hair distribution, sensory dermatomes and skin disease. *Bulletin of the Johns Hopkins Hospital* 70:442–59.

———. 1945. Lumbar sympathetic dermatomes in man determined by the electrical skin resis-tance method. *Journal of Neurophysiology* 8:323–38.

Richter, C. P., B. G. Woodruff, and B. C. Eaton. 1943. Hand and foot patterns of low electrical skin resistance: their anatomical and neurological significance. *Journal of Neurophysiology* 6:417–24.

Riley, L. H., Jr., and C. P. Richter. 1975. Uses of the electrical skin resistance method in the evaluation of patients with neck and upper extremity pain. *Johns Hopkins Medical Journal* 137:69–74.

Rogers, P. V., and C. P. Richter. 1948. Anatomical comparison between the adrenal glands of wild Norway, wild Alexandrine and domestic Norway rats. *Endocrinology* 42:46–55.

Schmidt, E. C. H., Jr., and C. P. Richter. 1941. Anatomic and behavior changes produced by partial hepatectomy in the rat. *Archives of Pathology* 31:483–88.

Tan, E. M., M. E. Hanson, and C. P. Richter. 1954. Swimming time of rats with relation to water temperature. *Federal Proceedings* 13:498.

Tower, S. S., and C. P. Richter. 1931. Injury and repair within the sympathetic nervous system. I. The preganglionic neurons. *Archives of Neurology and Psychiatry* 26:485–95.

———. 1932a. Injury and repair within the sympathetic nervous system. II. The postganglionic neurons. *Archives of Neurology and Psychiatry* I 28:1139–48.

———. 1932b. Injury and repair within the sympathetic nervous system. III. Evidence of activity of postganglionic sympathetic neurons independent of the central nervous system. *Archives of Neurology and Psychiatry* 28:1149–52.

Wang, G. H., and C. P. Richter. 1928. Action currents from the pad of the cat's foot produced by stimulation of the tuber cinereum. *Chinese Journal of Physiology* 2:279–84.

Wang, G. H., C. P. Richter, and A. F. Guttmacher. 1925. Activity studies on male castrated rats with ovarian transplants, and correlation of the activity with the histology of the grafts. *American Journal of Physiology* 73:581–99.

Whelan, F. G., and C. P. Richter. 1943. Electrical skin resistance technique used to map areas of skin affected by sympathectomy and by other surgical or functional factors. *Archives of Neurology and Psychiatry* 49:454–56.

Wilkins, L., and C. P. Richter. 1940. A great craving for salt by a child with corticoadrenal insufficiency. *JAMA* 114:866–68.

INDEX

Page numbers in italics refer to figures and tables.

Jay Schulkin received his Ph.D. from the University of Pennsylvania. He is a research professor of physiology and biophysics at the Georgetown University School of Medicine, senior research associate at the Clinical Neuroendocrinology Branch at the National Institute of Mental Health, and the director of research at the American College of Obstetricians and Gynecologists. Dr. Schulkin is the author of eight books, including *Sodium Hunger,* and the editor of three. His research interests include the neuroendocrine regulation of appetitive behavior and fear.